"DEVYANI"

And we, who are left, must grow old with the years,
knowing failure and heartache and blame,
while you stand on the hill with the wind in your hair,
Young and beautiful, always the same.

PREFACE TO THE FIRST EDITION

Neurology did not enjoy the status of a separate subspecialty in India till the early fifties. General physicians taught Neurology at both undergraduate and postgraduate levels. Even today, undergraduate students are not assigned rotations on neurology wards. Moreover, neurology is still not established as a speciality in many Indian medical colleges. We have been aware of the need for a textbook of neurology that would be useful to undergraduates and family physicians. The senior author has often found postgraduate students in Medicine lacking a sound knowledge of the fundamentals of neurology, and arraying vague concepts of common problems in clinical neurology.

This book introduces the subject of clinical neurology in a concise and lucid manner. There has been no attempt to include rare disease entities and references. However, in each chapter, detailed updated classification of diseases has been included for students desirous of further study. The aim has been to cover common problems in Neurology as they apply to the Indian subcontinent. Modern concepts of pain, migraine, and classification of seizures are emphasised. The eager student should be stimulated to read in depth, and some may be drawn to a career in neurology. The first two chapters deal with signs and symptoms. Certain clinical conditions such as migraine, coma, cerebro-vascular disease etc., are dealt with in depth in the initial chapters for the basic understanding and stressing the importance of good history taking and detailed examination. Later chapters describe specific clinical conditions in a crisp and simple manner. The authors have tried to limit the size of the book, so that it is inexpensive. Regrettably, this has led to fewer illustrations being included.

We would like to acknowledge the help rendered by Dr.N.H.Wadia and by many undergraduate medical students who gave us many useful suggestions. Special thanks are due to Mr. Ash A. Parekh who willingly acceded to our request to draw all illustrations and to Mrs. S.S.Patwardhan for the secretarial help.

An Introduction to

CLINICAL NEUROLOGY

By

Dr Anil D Desai

Senior Consultant Neurologist, Jaslok Hospital and
Medical Research Centre and Emeritus Consultant Neurologist
Bhatia General Hospital

And

Dr. Satish V Khadilkar

Honorary Neurologist, Bombay Hospital Institute of Medical
Sciences and Hon. Asst. Professor of Neurology, and Head Unit II,
Grant Medical College and J J Group of Hospitals, Mumbai.

With a foreword by

Prof. Robert C. Griggs
Prof. of Neurology,
University of Rochester School of Medicine
601, Elmuood Avenue,
Rochester, NY 14642.
Editor-In-Chief-'Neurology'
Journal of American Neurological Association

THE NATIONAL BOOK DEPOT
Opp. Wadia Children Hospital, Parel, Mumbai - 12.
Tel.: 2416 5274 / 2413 1362 • Fax: 2413 0877
e-mail:prachint@bom7.vsnl.net.in

Second Edition 2003

Published by
THE NATIONAL BOOK DEPOT
Opp. Wadia Children's Hospital, Parel, Mumbai-400012
Tel : 2416 5274 / 2413 1362. Fax : 2413 0877
E-mail : prachint@bom7.vsnl.net.in

ISBN : 81-87540-30-3

Price : Rs. 175/-

Printed by : Neel Graphics
Mobile : 98211 59155

PREFACE TO SECOND EDITION

Neurology is now established as a speciality in India and most of the major Universities in the country offer postgraduate degree in Neurology. Despite this there are very few practising Neurologists in the Country and the burden of treatment of Neurological disorders still needs to be shared by Internists and the Family physicians. We are fully aware that the First Edition of "Introduction to Clinical Neurology" was published in 1982 and major advances have occurred since then, hence the book needs a revision. The second author Dr. Bindu Desai, due to preoccupation, is unable to join in the venture; hence, Dr. Satish Khadilkar has condescended to help revise the book.

Dr.Mathew Menken, Chairman, Research Group on Medical Education, World Federation of Neurology, in an Editorial in British Medical Journal rightly states that do medical students, house officers and family physicians have confidence to diagnose and treat a patient with a neurological disorder. No! He states that Schon et al recently surveyed medical students, house officers and general practitioners and found that, compared with their knowledge of other organic diseases, their knowledge of neurological diseases was the poorest. It is this accepted fact, which has prompted the authors to undertake the revision of the book meant initially for this very purpose.

In last thirty years, the neurological pharmacopoeia has markedly increased in size. The clinical neurology needs revision as classification of major neurological disorders has changed due to vast advances in Molecular Biology. The disease pattern is also changing, for example, Syphilis and its complications are hardly seen now, instead AIDS virus is spreading in India, and this involves the nervous system as much as Syphilis. The format of the book has been maintained, but each chapter has been fully revised and modern advances have been incorporated.

Keeping in mind, the need of the undergraduate students, authors have decided to increase the size of the book, the number of illustrations and tables. However, the publishers have tried to keep the cost of the book as low as possible.

In conclusion we would like to quote Sir William Osler who said "To study the phenomenon of disease without books is to sail an uncharted sea, while to study books without patients is not to go to sea at all".

FOREWORD

The evaluation, the diagnosis, and the treatment of patients with neurological disease — the specialty of clinical neurology — have undergone astounding change in the past three decades. The advent of modern imaging techniques have with computerized tomographic and magnetic resonance imaging given us new insights in the relationship of structural abnormalities to CNS function. Functional imaging with positron emission tomography and magnetic resonance are even beginning to elucidate the pathogenesis of diseases invisible to the neuropathologist. Furthermore, molecular breakthroughs and the sequencing of the human genome have revolutionized diagnosis and given us entirely new categories of disease caused by mutations in previously unknown proteins: channelopathies, tau-opathies, torsinopathies, and nearly 50 others. In the process, we have learned that a "single" clinically-defined disease such as spinocerebellar degeneration can be caused by 20 or more gene lesions, hereditary spastic paraplegia by 15 or more.

The rapidity of change in the landscape of neurology and the taxonomy of disease might suggest that the practising physician needs to abandon the traditional, "old-fashioned" approach to patients based on clinical history and physical examination, especially the time-consuming task of the neurological assessments of special senses, of cognition, and of strength, coordination, sensation, and reflexes. Nothing could be further from the truth. Nowhere in medicine is there as great a need for clinical acumen and for practical experience with interviewing and examining patients and having well-developed powers of observation and interpretation of findings.

Introduction to Clinical Neurology, now entering its second edition, is written by clinical neurologists Anil D. Desai and Satish V. Khadilkar with the vast longitudinal experience in the careful assessment of the entire spectrum of neurological disorders. Teachers with long experience, they have seen the impact of new neurodiagnostic teachings and incorporated it into a wise approach to the patient. I can attest to the skills and expertise of Anil Desai having visited his hospital and seen patients with him — as well as seeing the skills of people he has trained in neurology. This book builds on the strengths of the authors as clinical scientists — emphasizing the neurological history and the clinical examination first and foremost, before proceeding to thoroughly up-to-date use of new technology to extend the clinical assessment and arrive at accurate diagnoses and appropriate treatment.

As one would hope, diseases that are of particular importance to the Indian subcontinent and its climatic and environmental characteristics receive appropriate emphasis. Thus, tuberculosis receives detailed consideration through practical examples — as always beginning with a clinical focus. This approach gives an authoritative volume that is appropriate for not only Indian physicians but for anyone who sees patients from India.

My own experience as a consultant neurologist for over three decades is that the practice of medicine in general, and most evidently in neurology, has succumbed to an over-reliance on neurodiagnostic studies. In my practice, over one-third of patients on whom I consult have been given a diagnosis based on a diagnostic study — but in fact have something entirely different causing their symptoms and disability. Obvious pathology on MRI or CT scan — small meningomas, focal atrophy, small infarcts, etc. — do not explain their headaches and many other symptoms. The EEG, EMG, muscle biopsy and even a molecular diagnostic test often mislead the unwary clinician. I have thus developed the absolute rule: "Never order a neurodiagnostic study until you have decided what the patient has based on your history and examination."

Introduction to Clinical Neurology by Anil D. Desai and Satish V. Khadilkar provides an excellent foundation for developing the clinical approach to diagnoses that will prepare physicians for the decades ahead.

Prof. Robert Griggs
Prof. of Neurology,
University of Rochester School of Medicine
Editor-In-Chief-'Neurology'

CONTENTS

CHAPTER I HISTORY

"Of Charcot it may be said with truth that he entered neurology in its infancy and left it at it's coming of age, largely nourished by his own contributions."

I S Wechsler

Foundations of Neurology can be met with in Egyptian papyrus, which contains the mention of Neurology and Neurosurgery. In India neurology was practised in Charak's time. Hippocratis had good knowledge of Epilepsy and traumatic neurology. Galen can be named as a father of experimental Neurology.

Clinical neurology flowered in the seventeenth century with two major centres in Europe dominating the field. The Hospital of the Salpetriere in Paris was converted from an asylum for infirm and abandoned old women into a world-renowned centre for research and training. Here Jean Martin Charcot (1825-1893) worked with enormous energy and an iron will founding a clinical neurology service that included Pierre Marie and Babinski amongst its students. The National Hospital for Nervous Diseases in London rivalled the Salpatriere in its prestige and distinguished faculty. John Hughling Jackson (1835-1911) and Sir William Gowers (1845-1915) laid the foundation of clinical neurology, their writings providing excellent reading even today. In the middle of the 18th century the technique of the neurological examination was gradually developed. In the twentieth century, the American subcontinent including Canada has provided quite a few scientist of the calibre of Charcot or Sir William Gowers such as Weir Mitchelle, Mills, Cushing and Penfield.

In 1931 Minkowski defined neurology as "science of the structure and of all actions of the nervous system in health and in disease, in man, and in animals and in foetus, the infantile and in the adult organism." While his pupil and collaborator Walshe in 1957 mentioned, "We pursue knowledge for a practical end - cure and prevention of disease, here nervous diseases". .

The art of history taking, always important in clinical medicine is crucial to neurology. A proper chronological account of the patient's symptoms, aid in the diagnosis. In India, the clinician has to deal with additional special problems. Illiteracy still abounds, superstitions are rampant and irrelevant problems like constipation are given undue importance, as patients still tend to return to the old *ayurvedic* principals of health. India is a multilingual nation and very often the physician and the patient do not share a common language. Moreover, multiple systems of medicine such as Ayurvedic and Homeopathic medicine are currently being practised. Much patience and practice are therefore required before a physician can obtain a history where not only is the 'chaff separated from the grain' but a proper time frame constructed which allows a probable diagnosis to be reached. For instance, a young man complains of progressive weakness of the right arm and leg. When questioned for other symptoms he mentions headaches but immediately adds that he had attributed them to 'overwork' and 'poor eyesight' and at times he may mention that his family physician felt that the headaches were related to his higher blood pressure. We are now aware that he also has headaches and poor vision; further inquiry reveals the headache preceded the visual problems by several months. The headaches began six months ago and were increasing in severity. Worse in the morning, increased by coughing and straining at stools, the headache was localized to left frontal region. Initially intermittent, it later became constant and was not relieved with analgesics. The visual problem began a month ago and was characterized as a difficulty in focusing objects with blurring of distant images. On the basis of this history we can suspect that the patient's problems are caused by a slow growing mass located in the left frontal region which has resulted in increased intra-cranial pressure, papilloedema and focal neurological deficit. Examination revealed early papilloedema and a mild right hemiparesis with increased tone and deep tendon reflexes. CAT scan examination revealed an intra-parenchymal mass, which at surgery was found to be a glioma.

The above case illustrates the importance of certain symptoms in neurological practice. Headache, vertigo, loss of consciousness, limb weakness and numbness are but a few of the common complaints. One has to know the chronological order in which the events occurred, to get an insight into the clinical course, whether the changes were sudden or gradual in onset and if the symptom has progressed or stabilized. We will now consider some of the symptoms commonly encountered in neurology, examine their pathophysiology and describe their characteristics.

PAIN

"But pain is perfect misery, the worst of evils, and excessive overturns All Patience".

John Milton, Paradise Lost, Book Six, 456-464.

Pain provoked by tissue damage due to accident, disease, and inflammation, consists of unpleasant sensory, emotional and mental experiences leading to psychological, behavioral and autonomic responses

Pain should be described in terms of its location, duration and character. Are their any precipitating or relieving factors? Does the pain tend to occur at any particular time of the day?

Research into the basic mechanisms of pain has expanded rapidly in the past few years. There has been exciting new discoveries and we shall cast a glance at the important ones. It is said that pain is not registered in the brain by neuronal activity of the specific pain pathways but is due to activity in several interacting neural system, each with its own specialized function.

The most accepted theory for conduction and control of pain at the spinal level is the "Gate control" theory. It states that over the dorsal root ganglionic neuron there is both inhibitory and excitatory control derived not only from dorsal horn neurons but also antero-lateral and ventral horn neurons. These neurons in turn receive inhibitory fibres, the large fibres from central cortical regions and the brain stem. Both these inhibitory fibres bifurcate and also have direct synapse with the dorsal root ganglionic neuron.

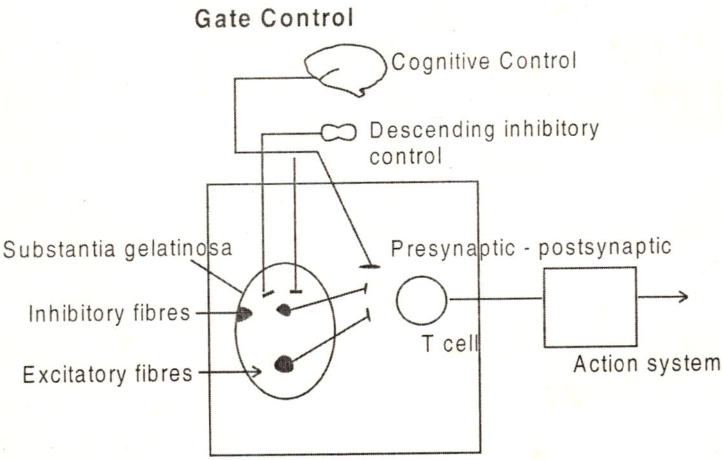

Fig 1.1. Excitatory and inhibitory fibres from substantia gelatinosa to the T cell (Transmission cell) and descending inhibitory and cortical control.

The conduction of an impulse in the afferent fibres of the cord to the spinal cells is modulated by the spinal gating mechanism. This mechanism is influenced by the relative amount of activity in large diameter and small diameter fibres. The large fibres tend to inhibit the transmission (close the gate) and the small tend to facilitate the transmission (open the gate). Descending stimuli from the brain via the fast large fibres also influences the gating mechanism.

Motivating, affective and cognitive aspects of pain pertain to the neural system beyond the gate. These involve interaction of projecting systems, namely neospino-thalamic (sensory-about location, intensity and duration) and paleospino-thalalmic (activates reticular and limbic structures provoking powerful motivational and aversive drives) with neocortical processes.

Dorsal root ganglion has a unipolar cell body from which the somatic sensory axon arises to establish connection with the sensory receptor peripherally and myelinated and unmyelinated axonal projections to the dorsal horn. (Table1.1) The unmyelinated fibres lie laterally at the root entry zone to form the Lissaur's tract in the cord, which ascend several millimetres to end in the dorsal horn.

They also establish connection with ventral, ventrolateral horn cells of the same segment and adjacent spinal segments. These connections provoke segmental nociceptive reflex response

Table 1.1

Nerve Fibre Types And Their Functions

Type	Diameter	Conduction Velocity	Function
A	16 μ	50 m/s	Largest, thickly myelinated; primary afferents for stretch reflex
	1-2 μ	15 m/s	Conduct 'FAST PAIN' which is sharp and well localised (e.g. sharp pinprick)
B	3 μ		These small myelinated fibres sub serve autonomic functions
C	1-2 μ	1 m/s	Very thin unmyelinated fibres conduct 'SLOW PAIN' which is poorly localised and persists after the stimulus is removed [pain in the traumatised limb]

The nociceptors serve as gatekeepers and survey peripheral information to be sent to the brain. They are of two types: the polymodal receptors which are under control of nerve growth factors and more specific receptors controlled by glial derived neurotropic factors. The nociceptive neurons carry specific receptors for the excitatory amino acids, capsaicin, ATP, prostaglandins, opiods, noradrenaline, neurotrophins, tachykinins and bradykinins with which they gather information from the tissue, to be conveyed to CNS. They also help CNS elicit different types of tissue conditions (various stages of inflammation, neuropathic injuries and regeneration, healing, metabolic disease), by having varying thresholds to the tissue breakdown and liberation of biochemical substances. The nociceptors also have special receptors for heat, cold, mechanical and chemical stimuli.

The nociceptive activity may be transient due to no significant tissue or nerve damage, reversible due to moderate damage with healing and regeneration within a few weeks, or irreversible due to persistent inflammation, tissue loss or neurogenic injury.

Sophisticated screening of the tissue conditions is carried out by nociceptors before it is finally made accessible to the CNS. These receptors are polymodal and mechano-receptors, hair endings, Meissner's corpuscles, Merkel's discs, Pacinian and Rufini corpuscles. For the impulse to be transmitted, it has to meet physiological, pharmacological and molecular threshold requirements of the terminal endings. The signal generating property change depending on whether the tissue is normal, inflamed, healing or irretrievably damaged. These changes trigger membrane receptors, ion channels, transporters - G-protein system, and also the second messenger cascade like cyclic nucleotides, calcium, phosphatidyl inositol, nitric oxide, eicosanoids, kinases, phosphatases, enzymatic arrays and axonally transported proteins.

The classification of pain should be clinically meaningful. It can be classified in various ways. It is classified according to its location, such as headaches, backache etc. It can also be classified according to the duration, such as acute, subacute or chronic. It is sometimes classified according to aetiology as somatogenic or psychogenic. The somatogenic pain is further divided into nociceptive and neuropathic. It can be classified according to the system such as myofascial, rheumatic, causalgic, neurogenic, vascular etc. The International Association for the study of Pain has suggested a multidimensional classification. This includes the region affected, system involved, aetiology (such as genetic, congenital, traumatic, infective, neoplastic, etc.), diagnostic, and differential diagnostic criteria. They have also suggested to consider associated features, aggravating and relieving factors, age, sex, sensitivity, quality, signs, laboratory findings, complications, social and physical disabilities in the total assessment of pain.

Table 1.2 lists the pain sensitive structures in the cranium.

Table 1.2

Pain Sensitive Structures

Cranial and Extracranial

1. Coverings of the skull
2. The skull and periosteum
3. Orbital contents.
4. Accessory nasal sinuses
5. Teeth and ears

Intracranial

1. Pia covering the circle of Willis and their major branches
2. Parietal dura along the base
3. Large venous sinuses
4. Falx and tentorium

Nerves

Above tentorium: Trigeminal
Below tentorium: Glossopharyngeal, Vagus and upper cervical roots

Note that the brain itself is not sensitive to pain but that pain occurs when any of the structures listed above are inflamed, stretched or dilated. The upper cervical roots supply the dura around foramen magnum. The character of pain varies according to cause. Pain due to inflamed dura is usually dull aching whilst pain secondary to the dilatation of blood vessels is throbbing in nature. The headache is throbbing in character and is either temporal or occipital, in migraine, hypertension, vascular tumours, post lumbar puncture, infective fevers and drug withdrawal. Eyestrain, sinusitis, and emotional tension cause tight band like sensations while the pain of meningitis and subarachnoid haemorrhage is described as steady and severe. Neuralgic pain is shooting in character.

As discussed above, the causative factors and pathogenesis needs attention but for relief of pain non-steroidal anti-inflammatory drugs are used. Use of morphine may have to be, resorted to, in severe cases. Recently, for relief of chronic intractable pain vagal nerve stimulation is used. More than 50 microampere inhibits pain by acting on the central pain processors via nucleus solitarius, nucleus raphe magnus, and nucleus coeruleus. The contralateral nerve to the origin of pain is stimulated.

HEADACHES

Headaches are classified as under:

Table 1.3

Classification of Headaches:

1. Migraine
   a) With aura - i) Hemiplegic ii) Basilar
   b) Without aura
2. Tension type Headaches
3. Cluster Headaches
4. Head trauma
5. Vascular disturbances
6. Intracranial pain
7. Substance withdrawal, hangover or lumbar puncture
8. Systemic and focal infection
9. Metabolic disturbances
10. Pain from cranium, sinuses, ENT, Eyes, Teeth etc.
11. Neuralgia - Trigeminal and Glossopharyngeal
12. Benign headaches due to cough, exertion, sex
13. Psychogenic
14. Unclassifiable

Headaches may be generalized or localized. The pain is referred to the fronto-temporal region in supratentorial tumours. In infratentorial lesions and meningitis the pain occurs in posterior auricular and occipital regions, whereas pain is referred to the vertex in sellar and parasellar lesions. The intensity of pain varies with the cause. It is mild in diseases of the eye with the exception of glaucoma, moderate in tension headaches or tumours and severe in meningitis, subarachnoid haemorrhage and migraine. *Psychogenic headaches* are usually described with extravagant epithets such as 'burning pain' 'inside feels as though it will burst' or so severe that the patient wants to bang his head against the wall. They may be either hysterical or tension headaches. The tension headaches are precipitated by anxiety; fatigue and apprehension while the hysterical headaches may result from a personality disorder. Hysterical headaches are present through out the day and night and are of many years' duration. Tension headaches are generally worst in the evening and tend to occur only during periods of emotional stress.

The pain of sinusitis is generalized and can be referred to the vertex if the sphenoid sinus is involved. Dull aching of mild to moderate intensity, it may be relieved by lying down with the diseased side up. When the frontal sinuses are involved pain occurs in the early morning and decreases as the day wears on. It is aggravated by bending down and emotional tension and relieved by analgesics.

Headaches caused by tumours are steady, dull aching and are worse in the early morning hours. Coughing, stooping or straining aggravates them. Of moderate intensity they are intermittent and do not interfere with sleep. *Headache due to meningitis* is present through out the day. Severe throbbing pain of a generalized nature occurs and the patient complains of stiffness of the neck.

MIGRAINE headaches are periodic with the interval between two attacks being variable. They may occur as often as twice a week or once every few months. Headaches can start early in life but generally appear around teens. They are more common in females. No social, intellectual or economical group is immune to migraine. A family history is often present. Migraine is precipitated by hunger, lack of sleep, exposure to sun, erratic mealtimes, acute stress, exercise, atmospheric pressure change, use of drugs, contraceptives and menstruation and in some by eating particular type of food such as chocolates, blue cheese, alcohol or yoghurt. Some patients avoid sour food or cold drinks. In majority, sleep usually relieves the pain.

The headache of common migraine is unilateral at the onset and becomes generalized as the headache progresses. The side on which the pain occurs may vary in each episode. However, patients complain of either right or left-sided pain.

Severe throbbing pain occurs, associated with photophobia, phonophobia, and nausea and vomiting. The patient likes to be alone in a quiet dark room. Vegetative symptoms like nausea, vomiting, fatigue, chills, thirst and oliguria may occur. There is no prodrome in common migraine, but the pain builds up gradually. In 1 to 17 % of patients with migraine, epilepsy may also be present. On the other hand reported frequency of migraine among patients with epilepsy is around 8 to 23 %.

Various theories have been put forward for the causation of a migraine attack.

Vascular theory: The aura and other neurological symptoms prior to headache have been thought to be due to vasospasm. This vasospasm leads to ischaemia, producing acidosis and which eventually dilates the pain sensitive blood vessels, the cause of throbbing pain of migraine. Methysurgide, a serotonin antagonist relieves migraine by regulating the calibre of the dilated vessels. It was hence thought that release of serotonin triggered the attack. However, this theory, which was once prevalent, does not explain the clinical features of aura. The auras progressively involve contiguous areas of the brain and hence are unlike the symptoms of acute ischemia caused by cerebro-vascular accidents.

Theory of spreading depression: In 1944 Leao described the spreading depression due to neuronal depolarisation and suppression of neural activity. The spread of depolarisation is explained by a double mechanism. The release of glutamate, the excitatory amino acid from dendrites depolarises adjacent neurones and this depolarisation then spreads as successive neurones are affected. Increase of extra cellular potassium also produces similar chain of events. Glutamate induced depolarisation is twice as fast as compared to potassium.

The scintillating figures are thought to be due to stimulation, a positive symptom while the scotoma a negative symptom due to suppression, the clinical counterpart of spreading depression. A diffusion-perfusion study by MRI has confirmed this regional hypoperfusion. However, it is now believed that the hypoperfusion seen in migraine aura is not due to ischemia but a part of primary neuronal dysfunction. The spreading endothelial constriction or spreading glial dysfunction either or both cause spreading neuronal dysfunction and consequent cerebral blood flow reduction. Further DC magnetoencephalography supports the occurrence of spreading depression during the migraine attack.

Neurogenic theory: The trigeminal nerve supplies nociceptive branches to extracranial arteries, meningeal tissues, dural arteries and sinuses. The electrical stimulation of trigeminal ganglion releases peptides, which promotes vasodilatation. During an attack of migraine, calcitonin gene related peptide is released into the jugular venous blood and this release is effectively blocked by Sumatriptan - an agonist of D subtype of 5-hydroxytryptamine1 ($5HT_1$) receptors of peripheral trigeminal nerve terminals located on the pain sensitive intra and extra-cranial vascular and meningeal structures. Moreover, Sumatriptan acting presynaptically blocks the neuropeptide mediated inflammatory response. It also induces contraction of the vessels, which helps relieve the headache. The 5 HT1D alpha-receptors are predominantly neural while 5HT1D beta receptors are mainly situated on the blood vessels.

Stimulation of sagital sinus leads to increase of calcitonin gene related peptide. The dihydroergotamine another 5HT1D agonist that passes the blood-brain barrier and binds to the dorsal raphe nuclei in the brain stem is also effective against acute migraine attack. It is observed that during an acute attack of migraine the Cerebral Blood Flow is greater in the medial brain stem structures as compared to pain free intervals. This increase in Cerebral Blood Flow (CBF) persists after the relief of pain. These areas are concerned with antinociceptive and intracerebral vascular control. This finding suggests that this increase in CBF is not related to pain but seems inherent to the migraine attack. This then suggests possibility of a brain stem generator for migraine.

The spreading depression most likely explains the migraine aura and the trigeminal and sagital sinus stimulation experiments explain the causation of migraine pain.

Patients with migraine have low excitability threshold of occipital cortical neurones suggesting that these neurones could be hyperexcitable during an attack of migraine.

Theory of Mitochondrial dysfunction: In syndrome of myopathy, epilepsy and lactic acidosis (MELA) due to tRNA Leu mutation, migraine-like attacks are seen. Two laboratories have documented evidence suggesting disordered cerebral metabolism due to mitochondrial defect. There is also evidence that there is systemic and brain magnesium deficiency in migraineurs. This magnesium deficiency can lead to abnormality of mitochondrial oxidative phosphorylation, which can then cause instability of neuronal polarisation. This then predisposes the brain for spreading depression.

Channelopathy: The gene for the Familial Hemiplegic Migraine is situated on chromosome 19p13.1. It also encodes the alpha1 subunit of brain specific voltage gated P-Q type neuronal calcium channel (CACNL1A4). In episodic ataxia there is disruption of the reading frame of the same gene. This then brings migraine alongside episodic ataxia, hyperkalemic periodic paralysis and episodic myotonias. Migraine is also associated with cerebral autosomal dominant arteriopathy with subcortical leucoencephalopathy and stroke (CADASIL) in which mutation of CACNL1A4 gene exists. CADASIL consists of recurring small deep infarcts, dementia and leucoencephalopathy. This mutation may affect presynaptic release of excitatory or inhibitory (serotonin) neurotransmitters leading to postsynaptic neuronal excitability.

In summary then, it can be said that an attack of migraine is a response of the brain and its blood vessels to some external triggering mechanism. This triggers the spreading depression, which as stated earlier is related to shift of extra cellular potassium and glutamate release. Calcium ion channel abnormality may explain neuronal hyperexcitability and propagation of depolarisation to the brain stem. This is then followed by activation of central noradrenergic and serotonergic systems, which modulate the pain. The disordered control of extrinsic and intrinsic circulation is secondary accompaniment of the attack.

Migraine is of various types. The regular attack of migraine without aura is called Common migraine. The attack with aura is called Classic migraine.

Hemiplegic migraine consists of episodic slowly progressive weakness with a march usually starting distally. There may be homolateral sensory loss. At times myoclonic jerks may occur. Expressive dysphasia may accompany an attack. Rarely fever, drowsiness, confusion and coma may occur. The gene is on chromosome 19p13.1, alpha 1 subunit of voltage gated P-Q neuronal calcium channel (CACNL1A4).

Basilar Migraine occurs around 20 years of age. It may have an aura of a field defect, dysarthria, vertigo, tinnitus, diminished hearing, diplopia, ataxia, bilateral paraesthesae or weakness or depressed level of consciousness. An emotional upset, stress, menstruation or a change in weather usually triggers it. Headaches are usually occipital. Seizures may accompany in 8 % of patients.

Ophthalmoplegic migraine mainly involves the 3rd and at times 6th cranial nerves. One has to rule out the presence of an intracranial anuerysm.

Management : Individual attack of migraine can either be relieved by administration of an analgesic like Aspirin, Paracetamol or other non-steroidal anti-inflammatory drugs either alone or in combination. It can also be relieved by 1 to 2 mg of Ergotamine tartrate used sublingually given at the onset of the headache. If there is no relief the dose can be repeated every 1/2 hour till 3 to 6 mg are administered. Ergot preparations should be avoided in peripheral vascular disease, coronary disease, pregnancy and thyrotoxicosis. Recently, migraine specific medication, an agonist of 5HT D1 has been introduced. It is believed to reverse the migraine pain mechanism. It stops the pain and relieves the associated symptoms. The drug *Sumatriptan* is available in the country and can be administered orally, parentally and nasally. It is hydrophilic and works peripherally, reducing vasodilatation and neurogenic inflammation. The dose varies from 25 to 300 mgm during an attack. Like ergot it is avoided in cardiovascular and cerebro-vascular disease. The side effects are paraesthesae, heaviness, flushing heat sensation, and intense sensation of tightness in throat and/or chest. In the latter situation the drug is to be avoided. Zolmitriptan, Naratriptan, Rizatriptan, Eletriptan (very effective) are available abroad. Few more like Fravatriptan and Almotriptan are undergoing clinical trials.

Prevention: It is important that a Migraineur understands his disease. He should have regular habits especially for sleep and food. He should avoid direct sunlight and wear dark glasses. Despite this if the attacks occur frequently, use of non-selective beta-blockers, Flunarizine and Amitryptiline, either singly or in combination for short periods of 3-6 months is indicated.

<u>CLUSTER HEADACHES:</u> occur almost six times more often in males as compared to females. They are usually seen around 3rd or 4th decades. The pain recurs for a week to a month almost every year or two. The excruciating, boring, knife like pain is usually unilateral and is periocular. There is associated conjunctival injection, lacrimation, rhinorrheoa and miosis due to paresis of the sympathetic nerve fibres in cavernous sinus. The pain usually lasts for few minutes to 3 hours. It may occur during sleep awakening the patient who may then start pacing the floor. It may also occur multiple times during the day. Alcohol and Nitroglycerine work as triggers. Inhalation of oxygen, Ergotamine nasal spray, 2% Lidocaine intranasal or subcutaneous injection of Sumatriptan helps to relieve the pain. For prevention, 60 mg of steroids is given daily for 2 weeks and then tapered. Verapramil 80 mg per day or Lithium carbonate 300 mg per day is also reported to be useful.

<u>HYPERTENSIVE HEADACHE</u> is said to be occipital in location. It is important to remember that headache is as common in hypertensives as in normotensives. Many hypertensives never have headaches and 'hypertension headache' has no diagnostic feature.

<u>SUBARACHNOID HAEMORRHAGE</u>: Severe unrelenting headache of sudden onset in a patient otherwise previously well should lead one to suspect *subarachnoid haemorrhage* secondary to an aneurysmal rupture. If the haemorrhage is large the patient gets a very severe headache accompanied by vomiting, convulsions, coma

or local neurological deficit. When there is small leakage of blood in the subarachnoid space on the other hand the headaches may be so mild as to be virtually ignored by the patient.

Almost 80 per cent of aneurysms are situated in the anterior half of circle of Willis and the rupture of aneurysm tends to produce frontal headaches, while occipital and nuchal pain often results from haemorrhage from posteriorly situated aneurysms. The sudden onset of a severe unrelenting headache accompanied by signs of meningeal irritation should alert the examiner to the possibility of a subarachnoid haemorrhage.

Headache following a *lumbar puncture, post-convulsion,* due to drug *withdrawal or hangover* is either deep dull aching or throbbing and is generalised. It increases by body effort, exertion or movement of the head.

NEURALGIC PAIN is usually shooting and sharp. It occurs in volleys and may be worst at night. The location of the pain will depend upon the nerve affected and may be over a part of the area supplied by that nerve or radical.

VOMITING secondary to intracranial causes such as tumour or meningitis is sudden, spasmodic, not associated with nausea and projectile in nature.

A variety of **VISUAL DISTURBANCES** occur in neurological disease. Diminution of vision occurs in the form of dark spots, which may be small or large, single or multiple and are known as scotomata. Quadrantic or hemianopic field defects of gradual onset do not usually cause the patient to complain of visual symptoms. Sometimes a history of a tendency to bump into objects on the affected side can be elicited. Rarely blindness in one eye goes unnoticed by the patient. Visual loss due to papilloedema begins with blurring of vision for distant objects. Total loss of vision occurs late in the course of the disease. Patients with well-developed papilloedema may have very brief obscuration of vision: 'grey outs' or 'black outs', dimming of vision usually involving one eye at a time for a few seconds and clearing completely. Visual loss in papillitis or retrobulbar neuritis is complete in a few hours to a day. Patients complain of pain on moving the eyes. Perimetric examination shows an enlarged blind spot in papilloedema with greater constriction to the colour red than to white. In retrobulbar neuritis there is a central scotoma and the constriction of vision is equal to all colours (Table 2.9, page 66).

DIPLOPIA or double vision is due to acquired weakness of one or more of the extraocular muscles. Monócular diplopia is rare and results from disorders of the crystalline lens or a detachment of the retina, or hysteria. Whenever a patient complains of double vision the following questions must be asked: 1) Are the images side by side, one on the top of the other or combination of the two or is the false image inclined inwards or outwards? If the images are side by side the lateral or medial rectus muscle is involved whereas if the images are one on top of the other the superior or inferior rectus must be affected. On the other hand if the false image is inclined then one of oblique muscle is affected. There are two main laws that govern diplopia: 1a) the separation of images is greatest when the eyes are moved in normal direction of action of the affected muscle, 1b) the false image is the farthest. 2) Has diplopia a diurnal variation, does it worsen as the day wares on. This is seen in myasthenia. Such a patient has no diplopia on awakening, but develops it as he gets up and starts functioning. It again improves if he closes the eyes for a while.

PTOSIS or drooping of the eyelid occurs when the lid obscures the pupillary margin. Ptosis may be unilateral or bilateral. Its causes are legion. Two muscles maintain normal eyelid tone: a) Mueller's muscle or the superior tarsalis, which is innervated by the sympathetic chain. b) The levator palpebrae superioris innervated by the oculomotor nerve. Therefore ptosis can result from a lesion anywhere along the course of the oculosympathetic pathway, which begins in the hypothalamus, descends to the thoracic spinal cord and then ascends via the sympathetic chain and the carotid artery to supply the globe. Ptosis can also result from a lesion of the mid-brain nucleus of the levator and along the course of the oculomotor nerve. In Marcus-Gunn phenomenon, eye closure occurs with chewing movement and the patient appears to be winking while eating. Inverted Marcus-Gunn phenomenon occurs in recovering facial palsy where on opening of the mouth the eyelid droops. The causes of Ptosis are listed in Table 1.4

Table 1.4

Causes Of Ptosis

Lesions in the muscle	: Myasthenia gravis Ocular myopathy Myotonic dystrophy	
Lesions of the eyelid	: Lid or orbital tumour (Haemangioma, dermoid) Eyelid infection	
Lesions of the sympathetic	: Horner's syndrome due to -	Syringomyelia Cervical rib Pancoast tumour Cavernous sinus lesion Tabes Reader's syndrome Cervical cord tumours
Lesions of the oculo-motor nerve	: Vascular occlusion: Benedict's or Weber's syndrome Basal meningitis - Pyogenic, tuberculous etc. Aneurysms of the internal carotid and posterior cerebral arteries Diabetes Polyneuritis cranialis Increased intracranial pressure- subdural haematoma Sphenoid ridge meningioma, Pituitary apoplexy	

INABILITY TO CLOSE THE EYES is secondary to weakness of the orbicularis oculi and lesions of the facial nerve. Weakness of the eye closure and opening together is almost always due to muscle pathology. The third and seventh nerves are rarely affected together as in mucormycosis of the orbit and polyneuritis cranialis.

DIFFICULTY IN PHONATION may be characterised as slurred speech, nasal twang, and hoarseness of voice or total aphonia. *Dysarthria and Slurred speech* is usually due to lesions involving the upper or lower motor neurones causing weakness of facial musculature. Slurred speech can also be due to cerebellar pathology. *Nasal voice* may be accompanied by nasal regurgitation and is due to unilateral or bilateral palatal weakness. Lesions of the recurrent laryngeal branch of the vagus nerve result in *hoarseness of voice*.

Total paralysis of both vagus nerves is not compatible with life.

DYSPHAGIA or difficulty in swallowing, results from weakness of the pharyngeal muscles. It may be due to lesions of the upper motor neurone as in 'pseudobulbar palsy', or of the lower motor neurone as in poliomyelitis or of the motor end plate as in myasthenia.

DIZZINESS is a common complaint. This word is employed by the patient to describe a variety of symptoms. It is essential that the examiner clarifies at the onset what the patient means when he complains of being dizzy. *Vertigo* is an illusion of movement that results from defects either in the peripheral or central nervous system. Ill-defined light-headedness or blackout is not to be confused with vertigo. In vertigo the patient feels either that he is moving around or that objects are rotating around him. Some authors define the former as subjective vertigo and the latter as objective vertigo but this division has little diagnostic value. Once you have determined that the patient has true vertigo, it is necessary to inquire into related problems such as pain or discharge from the ear, deafness or ringing sound in the ear/ears all suggesting middle or inner ear pathology. Numbness of the face or body, double vision, clumsiness of movement indicates brain-stem pathology. Epileptic vertigo is rare and is often followed by a period of unresponsiveness. Postural vertigo is brought on by change of posture and is generally secondary to labyrinthine disorders. Benign postural or positional vertigo is one example. It is thought to be due to concretion in the vestibular canals or utricle. It occurs in the middle age group. Females are more affected than males. It starts with an acute attack of vertigo with nausea and/or vomiting, lasting for few hours, followed by episodic positional vertigo of short duration. The full episode lasts for few days to a month. Positioning the head, as it occurs in certain head position, brings on the vertigo. There are no associated symptoms like tinnitus; deafness, sweating, pallor or drops in blood pressure like the Meniere's disease. The symptoms are mainly in the morning and they lessen as the day progresses. Usually, the vertigo does not occur unless the head is positioned. Benign positional vertigo has to be differentiated from vertigo due to vestibular neuronitis or labyrinthitis. There is a single attack of vertigo with vomiting and at times hearing impairment. The vertigo may last for few hours to a day. The episode may recur after a week or a month. The important differentiating point is that the movement of head brings on the vertigo but not positioning of the head as in benign positional vertigo. Vestibular exercises are recommended for prevention of recurrent attacks. Hyperventilation attacks are a common cause of vertigo especially in tense individuals. In Meniere's disease the vertigo is periodic, occurring at irregular intervals. It is common after the age of 30 years but can occur at any age. It affects males more than females and is often associated with migraine. The onset of vertigo is sudden and severe, the attack being accompanied by a sensation of fullness in the ear. Vomiting and severe nausea are prominent associated symptoms. Sweating, pallor, drop in blood pressure and even syncope can occur during an attack. Nystagmus is seen. Tinnitus and deafness in a single ear occurs later in the course of the disease. An individual attack lasts from a few hours to few days. Ataxia may persist for few days following the acute attack. Recurrent attacks are infrequent in the initial course of the disease, and may occur every few weeks or even after many months. As the frequency of attacks increases, there is increasing deafness with vertigo ceasing at the onset of total deafness. Early in the disease, the patient is unable to tolerate high-pitched sounds, which account for the "recruitment phenomenon". It is thought to be due to vasospasm and pathologic dilatation of the endolymphatic system in cochlea. This leads to hydrops of the membranous labyrinth. The acute attack is managed by advising bed rest. An attempt is made to find a neutral position of the head in which the vertigo stops. This is often unsuccessful. Prochlorperazine in the dose of 10 to 25 mg may be injected intramuscularly if the vertigo is severe. Since the cause of hydrops is not known, various measures have been advocated to prevent the attacks. Restriction of salt and fluid intake is recommended. Vasodilator drugs like nicotinic acid have been advocated. vestibular sedatives like Cinnarizine in a dose of 25 mg three times a day is helpful if the patient can tolerate the drug. The other sedatives are Meclizine (12.5 mg t.d.s.) and Betahistine (8-16 mg t.d.s.). If these measures do not help and the vertigo recurs often, various surgical procedures have been recommended such as section of the vestibular nerve or labyrinthectomy.

Post-traumatic vertigo persists for a week to months and is usually due to petechial haemorrhages in the labyrinth leading to serous labyrinthitis. Aminoglycosides like Streptomycin and Gentamycin produce persistent damage to the peripheral vestibular organ. They are secreted in the endolymph and they damage the hair cells due to their high concentration. Kanamycin, Tobramycin and Neomycin damage the auditory system. The damage to the vestibular end organ due to drugs like anticonvulsants, hypnotics, alcohol, antihypertensives, tranquillisers and analgesics is reversible and vertigo disappears on withdrawal of these drugs. Postural hypotension due to antihypertensives, diuretics and dopamine agonists cause vertigo on standing from sitting posture. Hypothyroid state is also known to produce vertigo. In central vertigo due to ischaemia, tumours, epilepsy, the symptoms are mild and are associated with other neuronal dysfunction symptoms.

The causes of vertigo are listed in Table 1.5

Table 1.5

Causes Of Vertigo

1. Benign positional vertigo
2. Vestibular neuronitis, Labyrinthitis,
3. Meniere's disease
4. Cerebello-pontine angle lesions (Acoustic neurinoma)
5. Head injury
6. Cerebro-vascular disease and brain stem ischaemic attacks
7. Hyperventilation syndrome
8. Drugs - aminoglycosides, streptomycin, salicylates etc.
9. Local bacterial infection, otosclerosis, fistula of labyrinth
10. Psychiatric disorders

The patients describe **MOTOR AND SENSORY DISTURBANCES** in a variety of terms. For example "heavy" and "numb" mean both weakness and loss of sensation. A weak limb feels heavy, as it is difficult to lift against gravity. Loss of sensibility including posterior-column sensation is often described as a limb being swollen and heavy. Limb weakness should be further localised into proximal, distal or global. Proximal weakness of the upper limb causes the patient to complain of difficulty in lifting loads or combing hair. The lower limb proximal weakness causes difficulty in climbing stairs. Patients with distal weakness complain that objects are inadvertently dropped from the hand, or the great toe often gets stubbed. Pain and paraesthesias accompany muscle weakness resulting from nerve root entrapment. Note whether or not there is atrophy, or any fasciculation. Is the muscle weakness symmetrical as in myopathy or asymmetrical as in poliomyelitis? Did the weakness come on suddenly, rapidly or gradually and is it progressive? The following terms are generally used to describe motor dysfunction. Weakness of a limb is described as "paresis" where as total paralysis of the limb is called "plegia". *Monoplegia* describes paralysis of one limb be it upper or lower limb, *hemiplegia* describes paralysis of one half of the body, *paraplegia* denotes paralysis of both legs whilst *quadriplegia* means paralysis of all four limbs. The term diplegia is used to describe paralysis of the legs that is secondary to cerebral pathology. It is commonly used to describe a paraplegia that occurs in cerebral palsy.

Bilateral lesions of the corticospinal tract above the medulla cause pseudobulbar palsy (Bulb=medulla). It results in emotional incontinence with pathological laughter and crying, hoarse, explosive speech, dysphagia, a spastic tongue and bilateral pyramidal tract signs such as hyperreflexia and spasticity. Jaw jerk is elicitable in pseudobulbar palsy. Sensory complaints are described as feeling of pins and needles – Paraesthesia, decreased sensation - hypoaesthesia or as an unpleasant sensation like burning pain - dysaesthesia. When sensory disturbances are due to peripheral neuropathy the sensory loss is distal in the areas of the hands and feet - described as "glove and stocking" distribution. In radicular lesions the pain and decreased sensation occurs in the area supplied by the affected nerve root. (Fig 4.2, page 157) Paraesthesia involving one limb or one half of the body is secondary to spino-thalamic tract dysfunction.

We have already described the pain of headaches and its related syndromes. Neuralgic, neuritic or radicular pain is severe, shooting and agonising pain that occurs in bouts in sciatica due to prolapsed intervertebral disc and is worst when patient is relaxed. A painful retro-orbital condition in which the eyes swell and there may be associated extraocular muscle palsies is the Tolosa-Hunt syndrome of painful ophthalmoplegia. It is more common in middle-aged females and responds well to steroids. Retro-orbital pain on movement of the eyes in any direction is usually due to retro-bulbar neuritis, affecting the optic nerve. In 80 per cent of these patients, the cause is multiple sclerosis. Causalgic pain is severe agonising burning pain following nerve injury, most commonly after injuries to the sciatic or median nerves.

A very important commonly encountered symptom is transient loss of consciousness. It occurs in *seizures and syncope*. The word syncope is derived from the Greek term 'synkope' meaning to cut or break. In syncope there is sudden cessation of brain function due to a transient reflex cerebral anoxia. The usual 'faint' is also known as a 'vasovagal' attack, and can occur with very little provocation. Minor trauma, severe pain, seeing unpleasant things such as pool of blood, prolonged standing in one position or emotional stress; each of these can lead to syncope. In syncope there is transient loss of consciousness. There is sudden fall in blood pressure with loss of vasomotor tone. Consciousness is regained rapidly if the patient is made to lie flat. A feeling of light-headedness, nausea, generalised weakness, visual blurring and slumping to the floor from upright position precedes syncopal attacks. The face is pale; the body bathed in sweat is cold and clammy. Rarely "convulsive syncope" occurs where there is brief limb jerking and sphincter incontinence. Some common causes of syncope are listed in Table 1.6.

Table 1.6

Causes Of Syncope

1. Postural hypotension due to any cause
2. Valsalva manoeuvre - cough
3. Micturition syncope
4. Hypersensitive carotid sinus.
5. Heart block - Stokes Adams attacks
6. Cardiac arrhythmias
7. Aortic stenosis
8. Hypovolemia

POSTURAL HYPOTENSION is defined as a fall in blood pressure, which occurs, on assuming the erect posture. Lying down relieves the symptoms. No agreement exists as to the normal range of postural changes in blood pressure. A consistent and persistent decrease of 25mm Hg or more in systolic pressure and 15 mm Hg or more in diastolic pressure substantiates a clinical diagnosis of postural or orthostatic hypotension. With hypersensitive carotid sinus wearing anything tight around the neck like a tie may induce syncope. In Stokes-Adams attacks the patient suddenly may fall heavily to the ground. Stokes-Adams attacks are generally due to third degree heart block or Atrio-ventricular block.

In generalised tonic clonic (grand mal) seizures there is loss of consciousness followed by jerking of the limbs: the eyeballs roll up, there is frothing at mouth, the patient may bite his tongue and be incontinent of urine or faeces. The seizure lasts about couple of minutes and is generally followed by a postictal period of confusion or sleepiness, which lasts up to at least a half-hour. The duration of spell, the sequence of events, and the postictal phase help differentiate the seizure from syncope. Though at times the difference is not clear. In such a case additional history and special diagnostic tests such, as a Holter monitor and electroencephalogram and serum prolactin levels are needed. These days video-telemetric EEG recording will help, but is expensive (See page 205). Gowers appropriately called this problem the "borderland of epilepsy".

Table 1.7

Differences Between Seizure And Syncope

	Seizure	**Syncope**
Cause	May be present	Present
Appearance	Normal or flushed	Pale, sweating
Aura	May be present	Absent
Convulsions	Present	Myoclonic jerks may occur
Tongue bite	May occur	Absent
Incontinence	May occur	Absent
Postictal	Confusion, weakness, sleep	Absent
	Todd's palsy (hemiparesis)	Absent
Recovery	Gradual	Fast
Prolactin levels	May be raised	Never raised

INVOLUNTARY MOVEMENTS: The involuntary movements involving the face, neck, trunk or limbs are sometimes encountered. The commonest facial involuntary movements are associated with chorea where facial grimacing is observed. The patient appears to be making faces and when asked to protrude the tongue he is unable to keep it steady; the tongue keeps wriggling and popping in and out of mouth. Details of each individual involuntary movement is as given below.

TARDIVE DYSKINESIA is a complication of psychotropic drug therapy. It can occur within hours of administration of the drugs, or in 50% of patients after 48 hours or within few days or longer. Coarse, repetitive and almost stereotype oro-facial movements occur, the patient making sounds that resemble chuckling or sucking. Respiratory, abdominal and pelvic muscles are sometimes affected. In children and young adults, trunk muscles may be involved with dystonic posturing producing opisthotonous or scoliosis. The dyskinesia worsens under emotional stress. Neuroleptics sensitise the dopamine receptors and disturb the dopamine-acetylcholine balance in the striatum. Tardive dyskinesia is difficult to treat. The offending drug is usually withdrawn. Baclofen, Valproate or Gabapentin help by increasing GABA. Clonidine has been found to be useful. Tetrabenazine and Reserpine are also useful drugs for relief. If nothing helps and the dyskinesia is troublesome to the patient then Botulinum toxin injections should be considered. Ultimately, stereotaxic surgery of thalamus may have to be resorted to if everything fails. FACIAL MYOKEMIA is characterised by involuntary unilateral fine continuous undulating movements of the facial muscles. It can occur at any age, persist for months or years and has been seen in multiple sclerosis, tumours of the brain stem and neurodegenerative disorders. Hemifacial spasms may occur as a complication of Bell's palsy, brain-stem lesions or may be idiopathic. Beginning as a flickering movement of the lower eyelid the movement may spread to involve the entire half of the face. Though benign the movements are very disturbing to the patient. MRI scan will help in the diagnosis of the causative lesion. The movements are suppressed by the use of tranquillisers at least in the initial stages. Botulinum toxin injections are most helpful. They have to be given by an experienced hand in the appropriate muscles. If nothing helps partial neurectomy of the branches of the facial nerve may be necessary to relieve the spasms.

TICS are sudden, stereotyped, complex, repetitive, normally coordinated but inappropriate movements, which can only be suppressed for a short period by an effort of will at the expense of increasing emotional tension. In some patients *facial tics* consisting of bilateral repetitive movements like blinking may occur. They usually begin either automatically or as a result of some extrinsic inciting factor or an intrinsic stimulus like conjunctivitis. They are then perpetuated as a compulsion after the original stimulus has long ceased to operate. Apart from facial tics, the *motor tics* may involve any musculature such as shrugging of shoulder or head jerking, or sniffing, or finger movements. The movement is sudden and brief. The tic can be either simple or complex. The complex tics are accompanied by impulsive, emotional behaviour such as, touching or making obscene gestures, involving a part of the body or multiple body regions. At times, brief inarticulate simple sounds such as grunting are produced by moving air through mouth or throat. Even complex speech like sounds are produced such as truncated words repetition of words (echolalia), repetition of the words produced by him (palilalia), or bringing out obscene words, (coprolalia). Even sensory tics have been described in which patients feel some sensations and respond to it by making sudden tightening, dystonic movement of the limb to suppress this unusual feeling. In 1885, George Albert Edourd Brutus Gille de la Tourrette described a syndrome, which predominantly affects males (ratio 3:1) and is found in all races. It is thought to be hereditary but risk of having affected children is low. The onset occurs before 18 years of age with tics as the predominant symptom. Varieties of tics occur, many times a day in bouts. Pallilalia, echolalia, coprolalia, echopraxia, and copropraxia occur in the course of the disease. Anxiety, stress and fatigue exacerbate the tics. Initially the children may have attention deficit disorder but the intelligence and affects are normal. The patients usually have obsessive-compulsive traits. It is thought to be due to abnormalities of serotonin metabolism in the brain. Haloperidol is the drug of choice, started as 0.25 mg and increased gradually up to 6-8 mg a day. The other drug called Clonidine is also worth a trial.

All patients need behavioural therapy.

TITUBATION is an involuntary movement of the neck muscles and is generally a symptom of a systemic degenerative disorder. The movement occurs in the form of head nodding at a rate of four to five per second.

TREMORS are rhythmic regular oscillating movements of face, limbs, trunk or head or part thereof. They wax and wane in amplitude from time to time, but the frequency does not change for a given patient. It is not a disease but a symptom or sign of a disease. Anxiety, fear, fright, serious competition in sports and fatigue exacerbate tremors. Bronchodilators, Lithium, Amphetamine and beta agonist like Terbutaline, Isoproterenol etc., Xanthines such as caffeine or withdrawal of alcohol or other addictive drugs, induce or exacerbate tremors. Tremors also occur in hyperthyroidism and hypoglycaemia. These are usually *enhanced physiological tremors*.

Essential familial tremors are coarse action tremors and are manifested when the arm is outstretched against gravity, or when person attempts to write or drink from a cup held in hand. They are absent in sleep. In 50 per cent of patients they are inherited. They rarely occur in children and occur mostly around 2nd to 6th decades. If they occur after 65 years of age, they are known as senile tremors. Tremor of the jaw is common in the elderly. There is no difference between familial, essential or senile tremors. Primidone in the dose of 25 to 50 mg twice daily or Propanalol 10 mg thrice daily helps relieve the tremors. Alcohol improves while fear and anxiety worsens the tremors. Rarely one requires carrying out stereotaxic thalamotomy or deep brain stimulation of *vim* nucleus of the thalamus.

Fine irregular tremors of the fingers are also seen in lesions of the anterior horn cells or its axons and in hereditary neuropathies. Hysterical or psychogenic tremors are irregular and coarse. They do not resemble any known type of tremors. The initial rest tremor of parkinsonism is described as slow pill-rolling tremor. It is characterised by flexion and extension of the fingers with abduction and adduction of thumb. It occurs at the rate of four to eight cycles per second and is present only when awake. Aggravated when the patient's attention is drawn to the limb and increased when the patient is emotionally disturbed, the tremor may come in the way of patient's activities such as eating and buttoning his clothes. In other diseases of the basal ganglia such as Wilson's disease the tremor may involve the proximal parts of the limb. This tremor is of large amplitude with regular movements of the upper limb, best seen when the shoulder is abducted and the elbow flexed. It resembles the wing flapping movements of a bird and hence is described as 'wing flapping tremor'. Rubral tremor is a rotatory type of tremor of the head or hands accompanied by random movements of the fingers and often an abnormal head posture. It is often present at rest and made worse by movement. Lesions of the cerebellar system (spino-cerebellar pathways, cerebellar efferent tracts or cerebellum itself) produce what are known as intention tremors. The tremor consists of increasing side-to-side oscillations when the limb reaches the end point. Postural contractions of axial muscles occur and hence, titubation of the head is seen.

ASTERIXIS is seen in renal and hepatic failure. It is not a true tremor as there is no alternate contraction of the agonist and antagonist muscles, but there is alternate loss and regaining of tone in these muscles.

BALLISM was initially described by Kussmaul in 1895 and is said to occur when the involuntary movements of the limbs are proximal, violent and flinging in character. Cases with generalised bilateral ballistic movements are relatively rare. They are described as hemiballismus when they involve one half of the body. Movements occur at both the girdles and have a rotatory component. In 2/3rd of cases face may be involved. Involvement of tongue and palate is rare. Patients can voluntarily control the movements for few seconds. They are less when the patient is relaxed and are absent in sleep but arousal increases the frequency. Ballistic movements are due to haemorrhage or infarct in the subthalamic nucleus (corpus Luysii). The subthalamic nucleus has inhibitory efferent connections with medial and lateral globus pallidus and excitatory efferent connections with substantia nigra pars reticulata. It also has small efferent connections with the cortex, ventral lateral and ventral anterior nucleus of the thalamus and putamen. Afferent fibres are received from lateral globus pallidus, broad area of frontal cortex and premotor cortex.

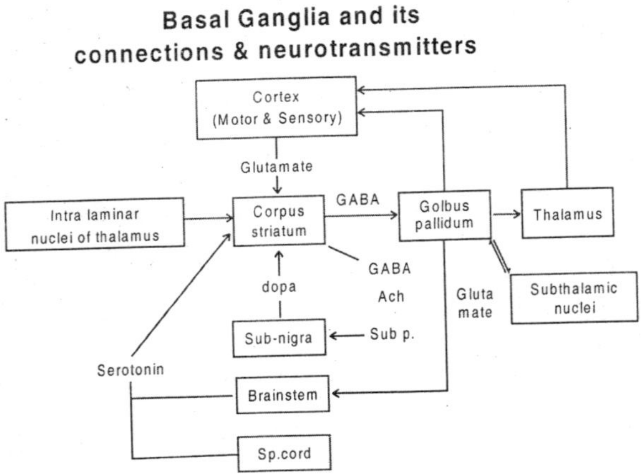

Fig1.2 Basal ganglia, its connections. and neurotransmitters.

The causes of hemibalismus are vascular - infarct and haemorrhage, mass lesion like tuberculoma or metastasis, AIDS, non-ketotic hyperglycaemia, encephalitis, neonatal anoxia, CNS lupus - antiphospholipid antibodies, and Behcet's disease. There are many drugs, which have been tried for treatment such as Chlorpromazine, Phenothiazines, Tetrabenazine, Reserpine, Progabide and Valproate.

CHOREA is a Greek word-meaning dance. At times the gait resembles a dance. It is a state of excessive, spontaneous movements, irregularly timed, non-repetitive, randomly distributed and abrupt in character. The movements are involuntary and involve the extremities both upper and lower, neck, trunk, face and respiratory muscles. Due to involvement of the latter grunting and other abnormal sounds are produced. It may vary in severity from restlessness, with mild intermittent exaggeration of gesture and expression involving the face, fidgety movements of the hands, and an unstable dance like gait to a continuous flow of disabling violent movements. When violent it can be confused with ballistic movements. However, the latter movements are larger, rotatory and involve mainly the proximal muscle groups such as shoulder and arm. On the other hand the athetotic movements are more sinuous, writhing, slower and more distal. Choreic movements hamper activities of daily living. In the initial stages the patient's relatives are unable to recognise the true nature of the condition and feel that the patient is mimicking or imitating someone. In very mild cases the movements can only be observed when the patient is asked to stretch the upper extremities. Hypotonia may accompany. Chorea may be unilateral or bilateral. Chorea may be hereditary or spontaneous. Sydenham's chorea occurs in the second decade of life and may be due to streptococcal infection. It may follow rheumatic fever. Rheumatic carditis may be associated with chorea but there is no neurological sequel. Recurrent attacks are known to occur in twenty per cent of cases. It is now thought to be due to autoimmune disorder with production of anticaudate and antisubthalamic nuclear antibodies. The specific antigen has not been identified. Chorea that occurs during pregnancy is known as chorea gravidarum. It can also occur following oral contraception. They are generally unilateral. Chorea is known to occur in polycythemia vera, in systemic lupus erythematosus, can be drug induced such as Levodopa, or can occur following head injury, brain tumour or cerebro-vascular accidents. The causes of hereditary chorea are Huntington's disease, acanthocytosis, Lesch-Nyhan disease (disturbance of uric acid metabolism), Hallervorden-Spatz disease (deposition of iron in basal ganglia), spino-cerebellar degeneration and Wilson's disease (disorder of copper metabolism). Haloperidol or Triperidol helps to control the choreic movements.

The excitatory action via D1 receptors from cortex on Gaba and substance P in striatum results in inhibition. Loss of dopaminergic innervation results in decreased direct and increased indirect pathway function which leads to excessive inhibition of the thalamus from globus pallidus interna and substantia nigra producing bradykinesia, increased tone etc. A shift in balance in the opposite direction i.e. increased direct and decreased indirect activity results in excess thalamo-cortical activity accounting for dyskinesia such as ballism, chorea or athetosis.

When chorea is associated with intellectual decline, following differential diagnosis needs to be considered.

Table 1.8

Chorea And Cognitive Decline

Huntington's disease	Neuroacanthocytosis
Hallarvorden-Spatz disease	Wilson's disease
Lesch-Nyhan syndrome	Mitochondrial disorders
Lysosomal storage diseases	Aminoacidurias
Hypoparathyroidism	Anoxic brain damage
Encephalitis	Systemic lupus erythematosus
Kernicterus	

ATHETOSIS is characterised by irregular, slow, forceful, writhing movements generally of the extremities, very often characterised by finger movements. The posture in athetosis is metaphorically described as a "policeman's hand". Kernicturus, anoxic disorders such as status marmoratus and toxic disorders such as carbon dioxide and carbon disulfide poisoning, Hallervorden-Spatz disease (Iron deposition in basal ganglia) usually cause generalised persistent athetosis. Persistent hemiathetosis can result due to cerebro-vascular accidents. Blepharospasm, writer's cramps spasmodic torticollis and orofacial or mandibular dystonias are classified as persistent segmental athetotic syndromes.

DYSTONIA: Oppenheim first used the term dystonia in 1911. Dystonic states are abnormal postures produced by slow sustained muscle contractions, which distort limbs or part of limbs, trunk, neck, face or mouth into characteristic postures. They may be distal (athetoid) proximal (torsion spasm) generalised, unilateral or focal. They occur at any age, beginning in childhood, adolescent period or adult age. Dystonic movements slow or rapid, are sustained at the height of movement, involve the same muscle groups and are usually repetitive and twisting. Typical dystonic movements include a hyperpronated forearm with a flexed wrist and extended fingers. The foot is inverted and plantar-flexed, the trunk curves to one side (scoliosis) or backward (lordosis), while the neck is rotated to one side (torticollis), or bent forwards (antecollis) or backwards (retrocollis). Dystonias are usually primary, or associated with features of parkinsonism, secondary or hereditary. Dystonic movements initially appear during active movement such as walking, later running and eventually at rest. In childhood idiopathic hereditary dystonia, the dystonic movement appears in one limb when used and gradually involves the entire body and eventually the dystonic posture persists. The locus of the dystonia gene is on chromosome 9p32-34.

The adult onset dystonias may remain focal or segmental. The dystonias disappear in sleep and are suppressed when the patient is resting. They may increase with fatigue and emotional stress. A variety of dystonia with diurnal fluctuations, absent in the morning and worsens as the day progresses, is responsive to treatment by small doses of levodopa. Some parkinsonian features may accompany this condition. It is due to mutation in the gene that codes for the enzyme, GTP cyclohydrolase 1.

Secondary dystonia is seen in association with hereditary diseases such as Wilson's disease. It can also be seen secondary to head trauma, encephalitis, and stroke or could be drug induced - anti-psychotic drugs.

Injection of Botulinum toxin for the treatment of segmental dystonia is a significant advance in the recent years (See page 92). Segmental dystonia involving the vocal cord, the eyelids, the neck, jaw and fingers (writer's cramps) can now be treated with Botulinum toxin injections. Levodopa, should initially be tried in the management of generalised dystonia. As stated earlier, some dystonias are dopa responsive. Trihexyphenidyl (Pacitane) in high doses up to 40 to 80 mg day help. Dry mouth, blurred vision and difficulty in micturition can be treated with Pyridostigmine or Prostigmine tablets and Pilocarpine eye drops. Baclofen, Clonazepam, Reserpine and Tetrabenazine are worth a trial either singly or in combinations. Rarely thalamotomy or pallidotomy may be resorted to. However, stereotaxic surgery should be reserved for patients who have undergone trial of all pharmacological agents and are markedly disabled.

<u>MYOCLONUS</u>: Friedreich first used the word myoclonus in 1881. Myoclonus is characterised by sudden shock-like contractions of a muscle or group of muscles. It may or may not be accompanied by

joint movements and may occur at rest or during action. It may be localised or generalised. It may be isolated and consist of repetitive rhythmic movements as in palatal or diaphragmatic myoclonus. It can be differentiated from other involuntary movements by few characteristics. A brief pause or silent period between jerks helps distinguish myoclonus from tremor. Choreiform movements are irregular. Tics can be voluntarily controlled for a period. Patient with myoclonus complaints, that he tends to drop things from his hands. It affects people physiologically at the onset of sleep - "sleep starts". It can be one of the manifestations of epilepsy and is seen in severe progressive brain disease like subacute sclerosing panencephalitis, and in storage disorders such as Tay-Sach's disease and neuronal ceroid lipofuscinosis or in post-anoxic encephalopathy of Lance-Adams that follows cardiac arrest. Other causes of myoclonus are, toxic or metabolic encephalopathy, Creutzfeldt-Jakob disease, late in the course of Alzheimer's disease, mitochondrial encephalomyopathy - MELAS (myopathy, encephalopathy, lactic acidosis and stroke-like episodes), MERRF (myoclonus, epilepsy and ragged red fibres) Lafora body disease and finally Unverricht-Lundborg disease. Myoclonus responds to Clonazepam, Valproate or Piracetam.

WILSON'S DISEASE: In 1912 Wilson described a clinical condition, that bears his eponym. It is a genetic disease with autosomal recessive inheritance, and the gene is located on chromosome 13, while the gene for coeruloplasmin, an alpha globulin deficient in Wilson's disease, is located on chromosome 3. Ninety-five per cent of copper is bound to this coeruloplasmin, hence not available for deposition in the tissues or renal excretion. In Wilson's disease since coeruloplasmin levels are low (less than 20 µG/dl), hence copper exists in free form and gets deposited in liver, kidneys and brain. However, it should be noted that the severity of Wilson's disease is not directly correlated to the levels of coeruloplasmin in the serum.

The disease can present at any age and may have either a psychiatric, neurological or hepatic presentation. Neurologically, it can present as poor scholastic performance, rigidity, tremors or dystonia. Signs of pyramidal tract involvement may accompany. It can also present as acute or chronic liver failure. The psychiatric presentation is, as schizophrenic or depressive illness. The renal defects are aminoacidurias and renal tubular acidosis. Renal rickets and osteomalacic myopathy may be seen secondary to renal tubular involvement. Golden brown, bronze or green coloured ring is seen in the cornea due to deposition of copper in Descemets membrane known as Keyser-Fleischer ring. Investigations reveal low levels of coeruloplasmin and excess of free copper in serum with increased excretion of copper in urine. Liver biopsy shows deposition of copper in liver cells. Penicillamine is the drug of choice, given in the dosage of 0.5 to 0.75 G/day to children and 1-4 G/day to adults. Oral pyridoxine is simultaneously administered. Trientin a copper chelating agent is now available and has no side effects. Administration of Zinc has also been tried to reduce copper absorption.

PARKINSON'S DISEASE: James Parkinson first described Parkinson's disease in 1817. In India, the disease begins before or around 50 years of age and has predilection for males. Most cases are sporadic and no specific etiological factor is known for the causation of this degenerative disease. Though, psychological trauma, head injury, exposure to pesticide, toluene and heavy metals, drinking well water in certain areas has all been blamed at one time or other. Majority of patients does not have a family history of the disease. Some familial cases have been described, with autosomal dominant inheritance. It is caused by a mutation in the gene for a protein found in nerve terminals, which is called Synuclein. Synuclein is also found in Lewy bodies found in parkinsonian brain. Several other gene defects have also been identified. Mutation of the gene for a protein called Parkin has been found. This protein helps to bind ubiquitiin to proteins. These proteins are then degraded by proteosome. Impairment of this pathway due to mutation leads to accumulation of damaged proteins, which ultimately causes cell death. Cigarette smoking is thought to reduce the risk for the development of parkinsonism. Clinical features similar to those of Parkinson's disease can also be seen in arteriosclerotic disease of the brain, following encephalitis, administration of Reserpine, Tetrabenazine or antipsychotic drugs, and carbon monoxide and manganese poisoning. Iron accumulation is known to occur in substantia nigra, which leads to oxidative stress. Nigral cells metabolise amines to form hydrogen peroxide, which in turn generates oxyradicals. The accumulation of oxyradicals can damage lipids, proteins and DNA. Oxyradicals can also be generated by combination of superoxide with nitric oxide. Impairment of mitochondria can occur due to oxidative stress or genetic defect leading to failure in oxidative metabolism of the cell and ultimately cell death. Excitotoxins also damage the cells. All these mechanisms ultimately lead to programmed cell death known as apoptosis.

Table 1.9

Acute Parkinsonism

Parkinsonism induced by drugs	Toxins causing parkinsonism
Anoxia	Vascular
Encephalitis	Injury
Central pontine myelinolysis	Extra pontine myelinolysis
Hydrocephalus	

Parkinson's disease is progressive. The pathology consists of degenerative changes in the pigmented cells of substantia nigra and the locus coeruleus. Almost 50 % of dopaminergic neurones in substantia nigra must be lost before signs of parkinsonism appear. What starts the process of degeneration is not known. Progression of the disease is thought to be due to three factors namely, auto-oxidation, excitotoxins and mitochondrial dysfunction. Once released, dopamine is destroyed at the synaptic cleft by enzyme monoamine oxidase. During this process hydrogen peroxide and free radicals of oxygen are released. Free radicals can damage the lipid membrane of the cell. Multiple mechanisms exist to destroy the free radicals, which may be deficient in parkisonism. This is the reason for introduction of Selegeline in the treatment of parkinsonism. It is said to stop further progress of the disease. But it has not stood the test of time. There are large excitatory inputs from the cortex to the basal ganglia (see Fig 1.2, page 28). The excitatory neurotransmitter like glutamate so released can be toxic to the dopaminergic nigrostriatal neurons. Amantadine used in the treatment of Parkinson's disease, is antagonist to the NMDA receptor and may prolong the survival of the patient. The third factor, which promotes progression, is the disordered function of mitochondrial complex 1 activity in the neurons of substantia nigra, leading to the failure of production of energy. Round hyaline bodies with a clear peripheral halo called Lewy bodies are seen in the cytoplasm of the pigmented nerve cells. There is also degeneration of the nerve cells in the pallidum with loss or thinning of myelin sheaths of fibres in ansa lenticularis and striopallidal and cortico-pallidal fibres. In late cases, minimal cortical atrophy has been reported. Biochemically, secretion of dopamine, a neurotransmitter is diminished in the striatum.

In 1980s drug addicts in California developed a synthetic heroin like substance - 1-methyl-4-phenyl-1,2,3,6-tetrahydropyridine (MPTP) which when injected induced parkinsonism bearing remarkable similarity to the naturally occurring parkinsonism. Animals exposed to this substance demonstrate loss of pigmented cells in substantia nigra with loss of dopamine in the striatum. Further, aged monkeys exposed to this substance develop Lewy bodies.

The disease may begin with the classical tremors, described earlier in the chapter or with rigidity. The tremors may start in one hand and progress to involve the lower limb on the same side and limbs on the opposite side within a few months to few years. Rigidity initially involves the proximal muscles causing muscle and joint pains. Patient may present with pain of frozen shoulder. Rigidity is of lead pipe or cogwheel type affecting both flexors and extensors equally. It spreads slowly to involve all four limbs. The tremor may exist, independent of rigidity. However, minimal slowness of movements (hypokinesia) will be demonstrable, and the patient may complain of altered handwriting. The writing becomes slow and the letters become small. Finally, in a small number of patients, the disease may begin with dragging of one foot and lack of arm swinging on walking.

The triad that allows the diagnosis of Parkinson's disease consists of tremor, rigidity and hypokinesia.

The facial expression of a parkinsonian patient is characteristically immobile, fixed with absence of blinking and a stare, giving an impression of a mask (mask like faces). Smile is slow to develop. The blink elicited by rhythmic tapping on the bridge of the nose continues indefinitely (Glabellar tap sign). The speech is usually low pitched and monotonous and the sentence may end in a mumble. Dysarthria gradually worsens and the speech may neither audible nor intelligible.

The patient is slow (bradykinesia) and has loss of dexterity in performing movements. He also has difficulty in initiating movements (akinesia), which at times, on meeting an obstacle while walking, makes the patient glued to the ground. It also leads to difficulty in writing, the handwritings becoming small (micrographia) and also produces difficulty in performing activities of daily living, such as buttoning, eating, tying shoe laces. The characteristic posture of parkinsonism develops later in the course of the disease. The patient stands with flexion of the trunk and knees. The neck is held rigidly, and the arms are adducted, bent at elbow, with flexion and adduction of all fingers.

Initially patient walks with slow shuffling steps. Due to postural dysequilibrium and impairment of righting reflexes, patient may have anteropulsion (festinent gait) or retropulsion, the former being common. In anteropulsion, the patient walks with quick shuffling steps giving an impression that he is about to fall forwards.

The autonomic disturbances such as excessive salivation, flushing of skin with sweating and constipation are usually present. Oculogyric crisis usually is seen in post-encephalitic parkinsonism. It consists of attacks of involuntary upward deviation of eyes with retraction of the upper lids.

The disease is slowly progressive without remission or exacerbation. Eventually the patient is bed-ridden though may live a normal span of life.

Treatment of parkinsonism with various drugs singly or in combinations is a state of art. Belladonna alkaloids are seldom used today. Anticholinegics such as Benzhexol hydrochloride or Trihexyphenidyl (Pacitane) is given in the dose of 2 mg three times a day and gradually raised to 12-15 mg per day. Two other anticholinergic drugs available in India are Orphenandrine hydrochloride and Procyclidine hydrochloride. The former is given in the dose of 50-150 mg a day and the latter in the dose of 20-30 mg per day in three or four divided doses. To get greater benefit of anticholinergic therapy, Amantidine in the dose of 200mg/day in two equally divided doses and Selegeline 5mg twice daily on empty stomach can be added. This will prolong the introduction of L-dopa therapy. The introduction of levodopa (L-dopa) in 1960s has revolutionized the treatment of Parkinson's disease reducing both the morbidity and mortality. Dopamine does not cross the blood brain barrier but L-dopa does. L-dopa is metabolised peripherally, hence to achieve greater concentration in the brain, carbidopa the peripheral dopa decarboxylase inhibitor is administered simultaneously with L-dopa. The side effects of dopa are chorea, tics, vivid dreams, nightmares, hallucinations and confusional states. Nausea and orthostatic hypotension are rare. The drug is usually given on full stomach. The non-vegetarian diet should only be taken at night as far as possible. Small doses of newer antipsychotics control early dyskinesias.

The early response of dopa therapy is dramatic and there is nearly complete resolution of symptoms. However, prolonged therapy produces response failure, dyskinesias and on-off effect. Within few years of introduction of L-dopa therapy one starts seeing the various complications of treatment with L-dopa. The abrupt transitions from an akinetic rigid state to normal motor functions or to hyperkinetic state is known as the on-off effect of L-dopa.

Dopamine receptor agonists are now used alone or in conjunction with L-dopa. They are of two types namely ergot derivatives and non-ergot derivative. They continue to provide relief after the beneficial effect of L-dopa is exhausted. Its simultaneous administration produces smoother response pattern. Half-life of Bromocriptine is 8 hours compared to half-life of L-dopa, which is only 4 hours. Bromocriptine is an ergot derivative and its early introduction in the treatment prevents emergence of response fluctuations. Pergolide a semisynthetic ergoline derivative is 10 times more potent than Bromocriptine. Pramipexole and Ropinerole are non-ergot selective dopa receptor agonists. The Ropinerole has affinity for D2 receptors and Pramipexole has affinity for both D2 and D3 receptors. They produce fewer dyskinesias as compared to

L-dopa. Tolcapone a catechol-o-methyl transferase (COMT) inhibitor enhances the effect of L-dopa by reducing its metabolism and hence its simultaneous administration with L-dopa reduces the requirements and dosage of L-dopa.

When tremors are not controlled by drug therapy and where the drug has produced involuntary movements stereotaxic surgery may be considered. It is again gaining grounds in the management of Parkinson's disease. Ventromedial pallidotomy is useful for reduction of dyskinesia. Bilateral pallidotomy is usually not advisable. Unilateral ventro-lateral thalamotomy is very useful for management of asymmetric tremors. High frequency deep brain stimulation of ventral intermediate thalamic nucleus relieves the symptoms of parkinsonism. Striatal implantation of dopamine rich neural grafts is under experimentation.

CHAPTER II EXAMINATION - HIGHER FUNCTIONS AND CRANIAL NERVES

EXAMINATION OF AN UNCONSCIOUS PATIENT

The higher functions of the central nervous system are examined in terms of level of consciousness, orientation in time, space and person, memory, speech including language, judgement and insight. The level of consciousness can vary from fully conscious state defined as a state in which there is awareness of the self and the environment, to the comatose state of unarousable unresponsiveness. States of altered consciousness include the confusional state where memory is faulty, but the person is oriented in space and time. Delirium is characterised by disorientation, agitation and perceptual disturbances with visual hallucinations. The patient is fearful, talks loudly, may ramble. He appears irritable and suspicious. He has attention deficit with inability to maintain stream of thought with any clarity. He is usually incoherent. There is disorganised thinking, and cognition is markedly defective due to memory deficit and language disorder. It has diurnal fluctuations with either normal behaviour or drowsy and quiet state or agitation with delusions and hallucinations. It occurs with general medical conditions like uraemia and hepatic disorders etc. Stupor implies a state of unresponsiveness in which patient can be aroused with great difficulty. In *akinetic mute* state the person is immobile and does not make any sounds or movements, though he is awake. It occurs in pseudo-bulbar palsy, post-traumatic state and late stages of parkinsonism. The terms such as obtundation, deeply stuporose, light coma, deep coma, make an accurate assessment of the level of consciousness difficult. In order to standardise the extent of neurological dysfunction; the Glasgow Coma Scale has been introduced. This scale relates "consciousness" to motor responses, verbal responses and eye opening. **COMA** is defined as no response to command, no comprehensible verbal response and no eye opening. In each of these categories the examiner determines the best response the patient can make to a set of standardised stimuli. The patient's response to the examiner's stimuli is assigned a number as outlined in Table 2.1 the highest total score is 14 and the lowest is three. The Glasgow coma scale has proved to be very helpful in assessing and in monitoring the level of dysfunction especially in patients with head injury.

Table 2.1

Glasgow Coma Scale

Examiner's test	Patient's response	Assigned score
Eye opening		
a) Spontaneous	Opens eyes on own	4
b) Speech	Opens eyes when asked to in a loud voice	3
c) Pain	Opens eyes when pinched	2
d) Pain	Does not open eyes with severe pain	1
Best motor response		
a) Commands	Follows commands	5
b) Pain	Pulls part of the body away when examiner pinches that part	4
c) Pain	Flexes body to pain	3
d) Pain	Body becomes rigid in an extended position when examiner pinches patient	2
e) Pain	Has no motor response to pain	1
Best verbal response		
a) Speech	carries on a conversation correctly and tells examiner where he is, who he is, and the month and year	5
b) Speech	Seems confused or disoriented	4
c) Speech	Intelligible articulation but speech is used only in an exclamatory or random way: sustained conversation not possible	3
d) Speech	Makes sound that examiner cannot comprehend	2
e) Speech	Makes no sound	1

The highest level of response to each command is recorded by circling the appropriate number and the three categories are totalled.

After ascertaining the Glasgow coma scale examine the fundus. Subhyaloid or preretinal haemorrhages may be seen in subarachnoid haemorrhage. The pupillary light reflex should be checked with a bright source. The reflex is preserved until the terminal stages in metabolic coma except when the coma is secondary to atropine or opiate overdose. In thalamic and diencephalic lesions the pupils are small but reactive. When the pupils are unequal and not reacting to light uncal herniation may have occurred. In tectal lesions the pupils are large, fixed and have a hippus. Hippus stands for alternating contraction and relaxation of the pupil. Pupils that are mid-positioned and fixed suggest a mid-brain lesion. In pontine lesion the pupils are very small but if examined under a magnifying glass the light reflex is usually present. Next examine the tone of the eyelids. Lift the eyelid and then release them. If the eyelid fails to close on either side it indicates involvement of the facial nerve on that side. Now test for blinking, either in response to light or threat. If blinking is absent on both sides it indicates pontine involvement. Check the corneal reflex with a stronger stimulus than would be used in an alert patient. Absence of the corneal reflex bilaterally is a grave sign implying absence of pontine function.

Observe the position of the eyes at rest. Are there any spontaneous movements? Are the eyes conjugate or dysconjugate? Roving eye movements are seen in comatose patients with an intact brain stem. The eyes move slowly from side to side. When the spontaneous eye movements are absent the doll's eye manoeuvre should be performed. Stand at the head end of the bed and briskly rotate the head from one side to the other. If the eyes move in a direction opposite to the head, the doll's eye response is present. If no eye movement can be elicited by this manoeuvre then caloric stimulation should be done. First check the auditory canal to make sure that the tympanic membrane is intact. Now elevate the bed thirty degrees above the horizontal so that the lateral semi-circular is now vertical. Irrigate the eardrum with ice-cold water. In a comatose patient the eyes will conjugately deviate towards the irrigated side and there may be a few irregular beats of nystagmus in the ipsilateral eye. Absence of eye movements even after caloric stimulation is a sign of severe brain stem dysfunction and is one of the signs of brain death. Since establishment of organ transplants, **BRAIN DEATH** can now be certified. The Indian Government has laid down following criteria: There are a few prerequisites:

1. There is absence of clinical brain function. The proximate cause is known and it is demonstrably irreversible.
2. Neuroimaging shows evidence of acute catastrophe
3. Complicating medical conditions like severe electrolyte imbalance, acid-base imbalance and endocrine dysfunction have been excluded.
4. There should be no history of drug intoxication
5. The core temperature should be = />32 degrees centigrade.

If the above prerequisites are met with than the following criteria also have to be adhered to before certifying brain death.

1. The patient is deeply comatose with total flaccidity of all four limbs and loss of all deep and superficial reflexes including pupillary, ocular, facial and pharyngeal.
2. There is no movement of any limb on deep painful stimuli and no grimacing of face.
3. The patient is unable to breathe on his own and is being supported by artificial ventilation.
4. The systolic blood pressure should be >/ = 90 mm of mercury. He should be euvolimic.
5. The caloric test carried out with ice-cold water as mentioned above shows no eye movements.
6. The spontaneous eye movements are absent with no doll's eye movements and pupils are dilated, fixed and non-reactive to bright source of light.
7. Finally, the blood gas studies (oxygen, carbon dioxide, pH, etc) are carried out prior to stoppage of artificial respiration. His pCo2 should =/> 40 mm and pO2 above 100 mm. Connect a pulse oximeter and deliver 100 % oxygen at 6 L/min intranasal or through the tracheal tube. The respirator is then disconnected for 8 minutes and blood gases measured. The carbon dioxide

saturation should show rise by >/= 60 mm of Hg., indicating absence of spontaneous respiration. During these 8 minutes the systolic blood pressure should not fall. The oximeter should not show oxygen desaturation. Finally, the pCo2 rise should not be only </= 20 mm, of Hg. The test is then repeated after some time. On the other hand if the test is positive, the patient can then be pronounced brain dead by a committee of four doctors - two neurologists, one treating physician and one the administrator of the institution where the patient is admitted. It is important to establish the diagnosis of brain death in institutions where organ transplants are performed.

Conjugate deviation of the eyes to one side or the other helps to localise the lesion. When there is a destructive lesion in one cerebral hemisphere, the eyes 'look ' at the lesion, that is they are deviated to the side of the lesion, the hemiplegia being on the opposite side. On the other hand, irritative lesions cause the eyes to deviate away from the affected hemisphere. In pontine lesions the eyes are deviated to the same side as the hemiplegia. When there is conjugate deviation of the eyes in the downward direction, it implies compression in the region of the dorsal brain stem. It is seen in thalamic haemorrhage. In the sign known as "bobbing", there is rapid downward movement of the eyes, with slow movement back to mid-position. This is also seen in thalamic lesions.

Motor function is tested in terms of tone and power. Raise each limb individually against gravity and let it fall. Sudden uninhibited flopping of the limb indicates that the limb is paralysed. Bend the leg at the knee and observe how the leg extends. If the leg extends gradually then there is no paralysis in that limb. If however the limb flops it implies paralysis on that side. Generalised hypotonia or flaccidity usually occurs in metabolic coma.

Observe the pattern of respiration. Cheyne-Stokes respiration occurs when there is a lesion at or above the diencephalon. The respiration waxes and wanes. There is a gradual build up and then a period of apnoea. Central neurogenic hyperventilation occurs in mid-brain lesion, ventral to the acqueduct of Sylvius or in the upper pons ventral to the fourth ventricle. There is fast regular breathing. Apneustic breathing occurs with middle and caudal pontine lesion and implies a prolonged period of apnoea at the height of full inspiration. Ataxic breathing or medullary breathing is irregular, ineffectual attempts at breathing. (Fig. 2.1) Cluster breathing occurs in lesion of lower pontine tegmental level. The breathing is irregular in frequency and amplitude with variable pauses. In increased intra-cranial pressure, there are one or two waxing breaths, followed by 2-4 rapid breaths and then 1-2 waning breaths. Finally, Kussmaul's breathing occurring with metabolic acidosis implies deep regular respiration.

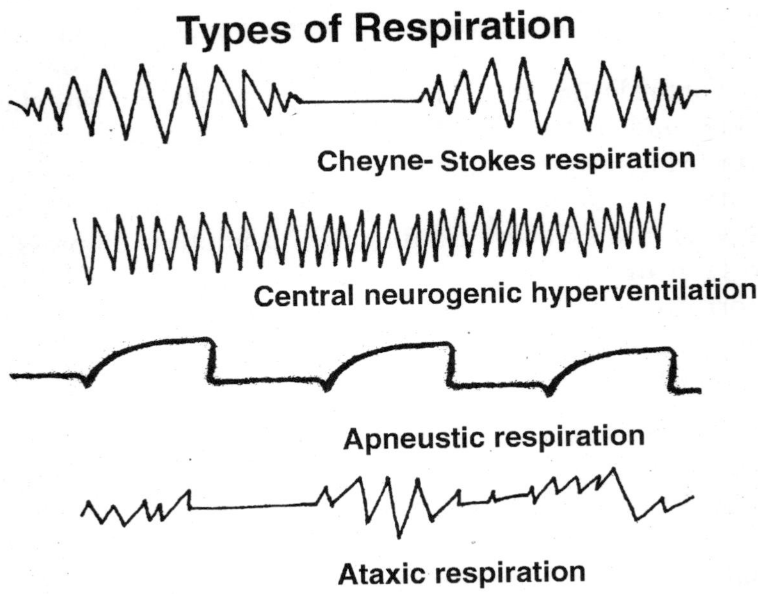

Fig 2.1 Various types of respirations.

The causes of coma are legion and can be divided into neurological causes and metabolic causes. The table below enumerates some of the common causes of coma.

Table 2.2

Causes Of Coma

I. Supratentorial Lesions	
i. Infarctions	
ii. Haemorrhage	
iii. Neoplasms:	Primary Secondary
iv. Trauma:	Extradural haematoma Subdural haematoma
v. Infections:	Encephalitis, Meningo-encephalitis Slow-virus diseases, Abscesses, Granulomas
vi. Seizures	
vii. Cerebral oedema	
II. Infratentorial Lesions	
i. Brainstem infarct	
ii. Brainstem haemorrhage	
iii. Brainstem tumour	
iv. Cerebellar haemorrhage	
v. Cerebellar abscess	
vi. Meningitis	
vii. Central pontine myelinolysis	
III. Metabolic Causes Of Coma	
i. Hypoxia	Pulmonary disease Decreased oxygen tension
ii. Ischemia:	Cardiac arrest Stokes-Adams syndrome Myocardial infarction & cardiac failure Carotid sinus hypersensitivity Low blood volume Hypertensive encephalopathy
iii. Hypoglycemia	
iv. Vitamin deficiencies	Wernicke's encephlopathy Pellagra
IV. Coma from diseases of other organs	
i. Hepatic coma	
ii. Uremic coma	
iii. CO_2 narcosis	
iv. Endocrine diseases	Symond's disease Myxoedema Addison's disease Cushing's disease Hyper and hypo-parathyroidism
v. Porphyria	

Cerebral infarction rarely presents as coma unless there is an associated cardiac or pulmonary complication or electrolyte imbalance. The coma in cerebral infarction is generally due to the occurrence of severe progressive cerebral oedema. The first indication that cerebral oedema is developing is a deterioration in the level of consciousness. The patient becomes dull and apathetic and soon is drowsy. A few become agitated. When coma ensues, the respiration becomes deep with yawning and intermittent pauses. The pupils are small, react to light and the doll's eye manoeuvre is incomplete.

A majority of intra-cerebral haemorrhages present with loss of consciousness. The haemorrhage may be secondary to a rupture of an arteriosclerotic vessel or it can be secondary to bleeding from an angioma or aneurysm. A majority of the patients with cerebral haemorrhage have hypertension, the bleeding generally occurring when the patient is awake. With the haemorrhage, the patient complains of severe headache and rapidly lapses into coma. In the initial stages a third nerve palsy may be seen because of uncal herniation. Later there is laboured respiration, a slow pulse and rising blood pressure. Finally pupils dilate, are mid-positioned and fixed. The respiration becomes irregular, the blood pressure starts to fall, and is soon unrecordable if there has been extensive haemorrhage with rupture into the ventricle, and there is a sudden profound coma, death may occur within minutes or hours because of ponto-medullary failure. Large haemorrhages could behave as described above but these days because of computerised tomography (CT scan examination), large number of small and even medium sized haemorrhages is detected, which in earlier days would have been labelled as infarctions.

A slowly progressive focal neurological deficit should arouse suspicion of a space-occupying lesion and modern investigative techniques should be employed to recognise the nature of the lesion. However, in certain instances coma can occur rapidly in a patient with supra-tentorial tumours. Some neoplasms tend to bleed. Glioblastoma multi forme, haemangioblastoma and oligodendroglioma are tumours that are known to have sudden haemorrhages into their substance. Coma could be post-ictal or due to non-convulsive status epilepticus. Coma can also occur if a tumour is displaced suddenly obstructing the CSF pathway as in the case of colloid cyst of the third ventricle. Multiple metastatic lesions in the brain can cause severe oedema, leading to early coma.

Pontine haemorrhage occurs in hypertensives with the bleed occurring during waking hours. The patient exhibits apneustic breathing and the pupils are pinpoint. The doll's eye manoeuvre may be absent. Flaccid quadriplegia with bilateral extensor plantar response may be seen. Examination of CSF reveals blood. When the hypothalamic centres for thermal regulations are involved there are disturbances involving temperature control and hyperthermia may develop a few hours after such a haemorrhage.

In coma secondary to brain stem infarction, generally, there is an antecedent history of transient ischaemic attacks. The patient would have previously complained of double vision, vertigo, difficulty with speech or numbness or heaviness of one or more limb. When coma ensues respiratory abnormalities occur, which include periodic breathing, spells of hyperventilation, or even gasping for breath. The pupils may be small or large and may not react to light. Hemiplegia or quadriplegia may occur and extensor plantar responses may be present. The patient may show decerebrate posturing on painful stimuli. When fully developed, the decerebrate posturing consists of opisthotonus, the arms are extended and hyperpronated, the legs are extended and the feet plantar flexed.

Brain stem tumours rarely cause coma. Patients with cerebellar haemorrhage develop coma suddenly. Some patients present with occipital headaches, vomiting, vertigo, deviation of the eyes to one side and/or ataxia of right or left-sided limbs or with a head tilt.

Extradural haematoma in supra-tentorial compartment is due to rupture of the middle meningeal artery. The middle meningeal artery is a branch of the external carotid artery. Many textbooks describe that this haematoma is generally associated with a so-called 'lucid interval' which actually is more often absent than present. Pupillary abnormalities precede the coma by a few hours. Initially the ipsilateral pupil is small because of parasympathetic irritation.

It then dilates because of parasympathetic paralysis and sympathetic overactivity. Finally it becomes mid-positioned and fixed. The triad of pupillary changes is known as Hutchinson's triad. Sometimes the pupil dilates on the same side as hemiplegia. This is known as Kernohan's notch phenomenon. It occurs because there has been contra-lateral damage as a result of the cerebral peduncle being injured along the free edge of the tentorium

Few patients with a chronic subdural haematoma may present with coma. They generally have history of headaches, confusion and problems with memory prior to development of coma. One of the classical phenomena of a chronic subdural is a day-to-day and hour-to-hour fluctuation in the level of consciousness.

Grey and white matter diseases rarely progress rapidly to coma and almost never cause a problem in the diagnosis of the coma.

With cardiac arrest and carbon monoxide poisoning consciousness is lost if the cerebral circulation stops longer than six minutes. Generalised convulsions may follow. The pupils are dilated; the plantars show bilateral extensor responses. If circulation is restored and consciousness returns within this short period of time then there may be no resulting neurological deficit. If the cardiac arrest lasts for more than four to six minutes the patient is left with substantial abnormal neurological residue.

Severe anaemia, myocardial infarction, congestive heart failure and pulmonary diseases lead to subacute or chronic hypoxia. The encephalopathy presents with confusion, disorientation and drowsiness. Progressive hypoxia leads to periodic breathing, small non-reactive pupils, myoclonus, decorticate rigidity and focal deficits.

Hypertensive encephalopathy occurs due to sudden rise of blood pressure in a known hypertensive patient. It presents with focal or generalised seizures, headaches, and vomiting with rapid progression into coma. Examination of fundus reveals papilloedema with exudates. Monoplegia or hemiplegia with unilateral or bilateral extensor plantar responses may also be present. The neuroimaging may show predominantly posterior white matter changes suggestive of white matter oedema (the posterior leukoencephelopathy syndrome). Good clinical recovery is the rule.

Hypoglycaemia occurs if the blood sugar drops below 40 milligrams and present with seizures or focal neurological signs. There is initial confusion and sometimes even a state of manic excitement. It is difficult to differentiate hypoglycaemic coma from other causes of metabolic coma; hence, blood for sugar examination should always be drawn in a case of coma prior to administration of intravenous glucose.

Wernicke's encephalopathy occurs more often than suspected. A patient with past history of alcoholism who has a poor nutritional status, and problems with memory, appears confused and disoriented on examination, should be carefully examined for nystagmus and oculomotor paralysis. If there is evidence of peripheral neuropathy then the diagnosis of Wernicke's encephalopathy is secure and intravenous thiamine should always be promptly administered. Proper identification and treatment of this condition is very important since the patient can lapse into coma, have a fall in blood pressure and even die. Pellagra is also often seen in our country because of nutritional deficiency. Skin changes and gastro-intestinal disturbances along with peripheral neuropathy are seen in a patient who will present with delirium and confusion. Pyridoxine deficiency is usually seen in infants and children. They present with tremors and/or seizures and lapse into coma. Patients on Isoniazide therapy and Hydralazine are also prone to develop pyridoxine deficiency.
Hepatic coma: When a patient with acute or chronic liver disease becomes apathetic and quiet, or becomes delirious and manic, incipient hepatic coma should be suspected. Coma may supervene after a few days or may occur rapidly within hours. When the patient is drowsy or even stuporose, the examination may show nystagmus, small pupils but reactive to light and asterixis - an involuntary movement of the hands, feet and sometimes the tongue. They appear like flapping wandering movements. As the coma deepens the asterixis disappears. In the deeper stages of coma decorticate or decerebrate posturing may develop with rigidity and extensor plantar responses. Patients in hepatic coma often hyperventilate because of alkalosis. Focal neurological signs like hemiplegia are rare and convulsions are even rarer. If focal neurological signs are present, the coma can be mistaken for a structural lesion of the brain stem.

However, doll's eye manoeuvre is present and the pupils show no abnormality. The serum ammonia is raised. The pCO_2 is low and the CSF is normal in hepatic coma. The electroencephalogram (EEG) is specific in the diagnosis and prognosis of hepatic coma. The EEG may show the classical anteriorly placed triphasic waves. These waves are transient and unless serial EEGs are done they may not be observed on a single EEG recording. In early coma the EEG will show bifrontal symmetrical slow activity and in deeper coma the background shows diffuse slowing in the delta range.

Uraemic coma: In uraemic coma, tetany, myokemic irritability, multifocal myoclonus and seizures are common. Focal neurological signs like monoplegia or hemiplegia may be present. In the early stages of coma asterixis may be seen. The tendon jerks are hyperactive and the plantar responses extensor. Acidotic breathing (Kussmaul's respiration), deep sighing inspiration with prolonged expiration may be present. Uraemic coma can be distinguished from hypertensive encephalopathy by clinical features. Blindness and papilloedema does not occur in uraemic coma but does occur in hypertensive encephalopathy. The CSF pressure is raised in uraemic coma. The fundi show exudates and haemorrhages in both uraemic coma and hypertensive encephalopathy but papilloedma does not occur in uraemic coma even though the CSF pressure is raised. Following features separate uraemic coma from other causes of metabolic coma. They are: a) presence of uraemic foetor (smell of amines); b) uraemic frost - a white powdery substance in skin; c) marked pallor; secondary to anaemia of chronic renal failure, d) changes in the nails - the moon of the nails expands so that the lower half of the nail is white.

Diabetic coma: Ketotic and non-ketotic diabetic acidosis generally develops in an uncontrolled or poorly treated diabetic patient. It may at times be the presenting symptom of diabetes. Generally there is a history of anorexia, nausea, and vomiting and abdominal pain. The patient may have mild elevation of temperature, the face is flushed and the skin dry. The respirations are deep and slow. The pupils may be large but react to light. No focal signs are present. The tendon reflexes are depressed. It is essential to differentiate diabetic coma from hypoglycaemic coma. Vomiting is absent in hypoglycaemic coma. The face is pale; the skin is moist and sweating may be excessive. There may be initial tremors and later focal neurological deficiency signs may be present. The non-ketotic coma may present as epilepsia partialis continua. The respirations in hypoglycaemic coma are shallow and rapid. The Table 2.3 below presents differentiating features in each of the metabolic coma.

Table 2.3

Differential Diagnosis Of Metabolic Coma

	Non-ketotic Hyperosmolar	**Hyperglycaemic**	**Hypoglycaemic**	**Hepatic**	**Uraemic**
Onset	slow (days)	Slow (in hours)	Rapid	Slow	Slow
Food	On food	On food	Off food	Loss of apetite	
Thirst	Marked	Marked	Absent	Absent	Absent
Hunger	Present	Absent	Marked	Absent	Absent
Vomit	Present	Present	Absent	Present	Present
Skin	Very dry	Dry	Moist	Jaundice	White frost
Face	Flushed	Flushed	Pale	Jaundice	Pale
Tremors	Absent	Absent	Present	Asterixis	Asterixis
CNS signs	Absent	Absent	Present	Absent	Focal Present
Respirat- -ions	Rapid	Deep, slow	shallow, rapid	Hyperve- ntilate	Foetor
Acidosis	Mild/absent	Present	Absent	Alkalosis	Present
EEG	Slow	Slow	Low voltage	Characte- ristic slow	Slow

Barbiturate and other sedative drug poisoning: During the drowsy state nystagmus, ataxia and dysarthria are present. As the coma deepens the doll's eye manoeuvre fails to show eye movements, the pupils remain small but are reactive to light and caloric testing of the ears shows depressed or absent response. There is generalised flaccidity, the deep tendon jerks are hypoactive or absent, respirations are slow and the blood pressure with deepening coma falls.

EXAMINATION OF AN ALERT PATIENT

The assessment of an alert individual begins with tests of cognitive function. Many specific tests of cognition are usually unnecessary in routine neurological examination. If the patient is able to give a lucid detailed account of his illness in a chronological order, it clearly indicates that he has normal memory and orientation. Mood and attention span can also be assessed during the interview. Gestures, grimaces, tics and other involuntary movements may be observed. Whilst the patient narrates the history, closely observe whether there is any thought disorder. Delusions of grandeur, hallucinations of taste or smell may be mentioned. The patient's insight and judgement can be assessed by his/her attitude towards the present illness, and the resultant financial and emotional strains that result from the illness.

Asking the patient to recall some recent events such as the date of admission to hospital further assesses memory. The general information and past memory can be tested by asking the patient to recall milestones in Indian history such as the year of India's independence. If the patient is illiterate ask him to recall past events in his own life, such as the ages of his children etc.

Tests for recent memory include the digit span test in which the patient repeats a series of numbers forwards and backwards. Begin by asking the patient to repeat three to four digits. A normal person will be able to repeat 7 digits forwards and 4 digits backwards. Simple calculation such as subtracting 7 from a 100 is then done. The patient is asked to subtract 7 from 100 and then continue to subtract 7 from the result in a serial manner. Tests for cognitive function are especially important in dementia and parietal lobe lesions.

The relationship between language and brain was first recognised in the 19thcentury. Phrenologists associated bony protrusions in the skull to the enlargement of the brain underneath. They assigned the development of various capabilities to these enlargements. They assigned language to the frontal poles. It was Paul Broca a French physician and anthropologist who observed lesions in left third frontal convolution, producing speech difficulty. He suggested that in patients who use right hand for writing, the left hemisphere control the language production and vice versa. However, this has not stood the test of time. It is now noted that the left hemisphere is dominant in 70 % of people who use left hand for writing and in all those who use right hand for writing. Wernicke found lesions posteriorly, in left superior temporal lobe, in patients who had severe impairment of comprehension of language. He called this area as "auditory word storage" area. This is necessary for production and comprehension of speech. He also hypothesised that there is a connecting tract (arcuate fibres) between this area and the area described by Broca. Lesions of this tract, in the supramarginal gyrus and areas deep in the sensory cortex in parietal lobe causes speech production disorder with disorder of repetition but intact comprehension

LANGUAGE is defined as the art of communication of ideas and thoughts by means of symbols either written or spoken. Disorders of language due to lesions of the cerebral speech areas are known as aphasias. Disorder of spoken speech due to affection of the peripheral mechanism of speech production is known as dysarthria. In aphonia, vocalisation is absent due to laryngeal involvement but the patient retains the ability to understand both spoken and written language.

Table 2.4

Dysarthria

Extra pyramidal	Parkinson's disease	Monotonous mumbling Slow
Cerebellar	-	Staccato, scanning
Upper motor neurone	Motor neurone disease Multi infarct state	Spastic (like pebbles in mouth
Lower motor neurone	Myasthenia gravis	Nasal, poor definition

For clinical purposes it is convenient to divide aphasia into fluent and non-fluent depending on the characteristics of language disorder. (Fig. 2.1) The aphasia is also dependent on the site of the lesion that could be either anterior or posterior to the Rolandic fissure.

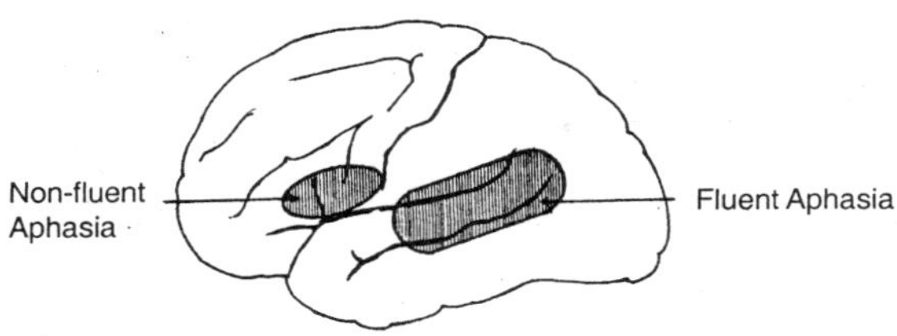

Fig 2.1 Lesions producing fluent and non-fluent aphasias

Patient's inability to repeat spoken speech is known as Conduction aphasia (Fig.2.2)

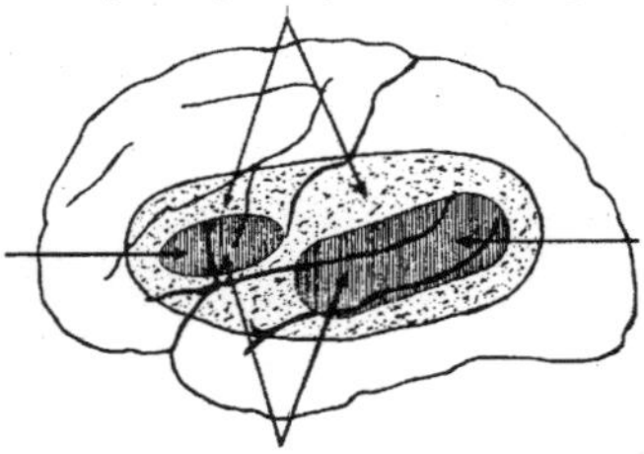

Fig 2.2 Area showing inability to repeat spoken speech (conduction aphasia)

Table 2.5 classifies the clinical varieties of aphasia.

Table 2.5

Clinical Varieties Of Aphasia

A. Aphasia with repetition disturbance

1. Global.
2. Broca's aphasia
3. Wernicke's aphasia
4. Conduction aphasia

B. Aphasia without repetition disturbance

1. Transcortical mixed aphasia
2. Transcortical motor aphasia
3. Transcortical sensory aphasia
4. Anomic aphasia

C. Disturbance primarily affecting reading and writing

1. Alexia with agraphia

D. Syndromes with disturbance of a single language modality

1. Alexia without agraphia
2. Aphemia
3. Pure word deafness

E. Non-aphasic misnaming

BROCA'S APHASIA is a non-fluent aphasia, which manifests as stammering in its minor form, and as short, hesitant, telegraphic speech in its major form. Speech output is reduced to 5-10 words per minute. Even these words are enunciated with great effort, the patient resorting to facial grimacing, body movements and gesturing to convey his thoughts or intentions. *Dysprosody* describes the unmelodic, arrhythmic, slurred speech of a non-fluent aphasic. In its most severe form the patient's vocabulary may consist of a single word, which is used repeatedly and incorrectly. The lesion is in the posterior frontal lobe. In lesions of Broca's area there is inability to repeat spoken speech. Comprehension of spoken and written speech is preserved.

<u>In fluent aphasia</u>, also known as <u>sensory aphasia</u> or **WERNICKE'S APHASIA** the word output is higher than normal at 100-200 words per minute. They come out effortlessly, with correct intonation and rhythm. However, there may be pauses during speech with words inserted randomly producing no meaningful speech. Paraphasia - generation of words by substitution of syllables leading to errors in word production. This could be either verbal where in there is substitution of words such as doctor for nurse or horse for house or literal (phonemic neologism) doctin for doctor, knows what the word sounds like but fails at attempts. Paragrammatism stands for faulty grammar leading to simplification of sentence structure by omission of articles, prepositions and auxiliary words and mistakes in tense. Both are present. Depending upon the extent of lesion the patient may have only babbling or baby speech. Understanding of spoken and written language is also affected. Patient is unable to repeat spoken speech. In conduction aphasia both paraphasia and paragrammatism are more pronounced.

GLOBAL OR CENTRAL APHASIA, there is lack of any word output, except some sounds. Patient is unable to understand simple commands and spoken speech. The entire mechanism of language formation is deranged. The lesion is extensive, involving the frontal, parietal and temporal speech areas on dominant side. Block of middle cerebral artery on left side or a tumour usually leads to this type of aphasia.

TRANSCORTICAL SENSORY OR MOTOR APHASIA is similar to Wernicke's and Broca's aphasia respectively except their ability to repeat spoken speech is preserved.

In **PURE WORD DEAFNESS** the reception and understanding of spoken speech is affected with intact comprehension of written language. This form of aphasia is extremely rare, the lesion being in dominant Heschl's gyrus. In pure word blindness on the other hand there is difficulty in comprehension of written language with preservation of the understanding of spoken speech. The lesion is in the parieto-occipital region. *Alexia* means an inability to understand and read written language. In its minor form it is known as dyslexia. In <u>developmental dyslexia</u> a child has difficulty in reading at an early age. They make mistakes in spellings while writing and at times write, mirror images of letters B, D, P, R etc. They may also have right-left disorientation and at times difficulty in recognising colours. In *alexia without agraphia* there is inability to read, whilst the ability to write is unaffected. The lesion is in dominant occipital lobe with involvement of the splenium of corpus callosum.

In **NOMINAL APHASIA** the patient's speech appears normal, comprehension of spoken and written speech is also normal, but there is difficulty in naming objects. For instance when shown a pen, the patient calls it a 'nab' or 'nen' but when offered the correct name he immediately accepts it. On being shown another object he persists with the word 'pen' though he is aware that he is wrong. This is known as perseveration. The lesion is said to be localisable in the dominant angular gyrus. The nominal aphasia is more often not localisable, being seen even in aphasia due to thalamic lesions. (Fig. 2.3)

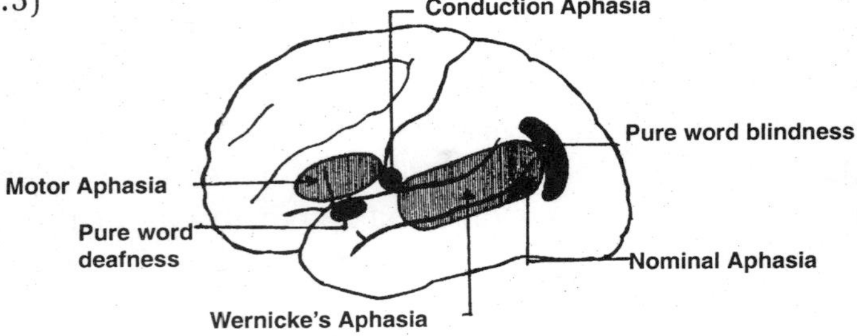

Fig: 2.3 Schematic diagram showing lesions producing different types of aphasia

An aphasic patient should first be observed carefully. Note the word output and rhythm. Ask the patient to repeat, read and write. Check to see whether comprehension is impaired or not. Detailed aphasic testing requires patience and skill and may only be completed after several sessions.

Table 2.6

Characteristics of Different Aphasias

Type of aphasia	Speech	Naming Repetition	Sentence Production	Word Comprehension	Sentence
Global	No Output	Absent	Nil	Nil	Nil, Unable
Broca	Non- Fluent	Impaired	Telegraphic	Impaired	Impaired Unable
Wernicke	Fluent	Impaired	Paraphasia Paragram- matism	Present	Impaired Unable
Conduction	Fluent- Variable	Impaired	Paraphasia	"	Present Unable
Transcortical sensory	" Present	" But empty	Structured	Impaired	Impaired
Transcortical Motor	Non-fluent present	Variable	Telegraphic	"	"
Anomia	Fluent present	Impaired	Present Circumlocutory	"	Present

The classification of aphasias helps the clinician to localise the lesion but with limited accuracy, however, it helps in understanding the formation of language. It also helps in prognosis but again to a limited extent. Hence, the findings of the language disturbance have to be correlated with other abnormal neurological findings to finally localise the lesion.

CRANIAL NERVES

OLFACTORY NERVE (First cranial nerve): The olfactory receptor cells are bipolar sensory neurones, which has a limited life on an average of 30 days. The dendritic knobs bearing cilia extend to the mucous membrane of the nasal cavity. The thin unmyelinated axons travel in bundles through the cribriform plate into the olfactory bulbs situated at the base of the anterior cranial fossa underneath the frontal lobes. Second relay fibres arise from the bulb and proceed caudally as olfactory tract and end in uncus, hippocampal gyri, amygdaloid complex and entorhinal cortex, which are the cortical centres for smell. The environmental toxins and viruses can get access to the brain through this pathway. Functional MRI detects activation of these and other areas of the frontal cortex and cingulate gyri on olfactory stimulation. The olfactory stimulation increases cerebral blood flow in the region of the pyriform cortex. Excision of the pyriform cortex during temporal lobectomy affects odour identification and also impairs odour reception memory, while sparing the ability to detect the odorants.

The nasal passages are innervated by the dendritic knobs of the olfactory receptor cells and also by the free endings of the trigeminal nerve. The latter respond to large variety of volatile chemical stimuli. The olfactory filaments respond to the chemical stimuli at lower concentrations with greater selectivity than the trigeminal endings and are responsible for recognising odorous substances. It must be remembered that in anosmia the capacity to distinguish odours is lost but response to nasal mucous membrane stimulation and irritation is preserved. In parosmia or dysosmia there is distortion of the sense of smell.

To check the sense of smell the patient is asked to close his eyes and recognise different smells offered to him near the nostril. One nostril is tested at one time, the other nostril being blocked by the examiner's finger. Perfumes, camphor, menthol, coffee etc. are held near the open nostril and the patient is asked to inhale slowly and identify the substances. The sense of smell may be affected due to local lesions of the nasal mucosa as well as lesions of the olfactory nerves and its pathways. Head injury and olfactory groove meningioma are the commonest neurological causes of the loss of sense of smell. Head injury may result in an altered sense of smell called *parosmia* where strong odours acquire an unpleasant quality. Hallucinations of smell arise in some types of epilepsy and encephalitis. The odour felt is usually strong and foul. The epileptiform discharge arises in the uncinate region of the temporal lobe.

THE OPTIC NERVE (Second Cranial Nerve) The fibres of the optic nerve arise from the retina and exit at the optic nerve head where they acquire a myelin sheath. The optic nerve head or optic disc appears as a pinkish circular disk on direct opthalmoscopic (fundoscopic) examination. There is a depression in the centre of the disc known as optic cup through which the artery enters and the vein leaves the eye. The nerve proceeds to enter the cranial cavity through the optic foramen of the sphenoid bone. Both optic nerves then proceed caudally and medially to meet and form the chiasm. Fibres from the nasal half of both retinas decussate and proceed in the contralateral optic tract. The fibres from temporal half of both retinas proceed without decussation in the ipsilateral optic tract. Crossed fibres are 53% and uncrossed 47%. The optic tract thus formed travels posteriorly to the lateral geniculate body that has six layers of cells and is a part of the thalamus. Ipsilateral fibres end in layers 2,3, and 5 and contralateral in layers 1,4 and 6. Layers 1 and 2 are magnocellular concerned with detection of movements and dynamic form of perception.

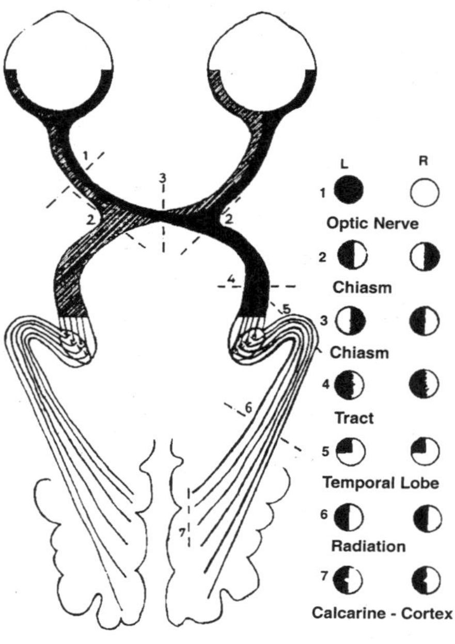

Fig 2.4 Depicts optic pathways and lesions at various levels

Fibres subserving the pupillary light reflex do not synapse in the lateral geniculate body and leave the visual pathway to travel towards the quadrigeminal plate of the midbrain. This therefore explains preservation of light reflex after lesion of visual cortex producing cortical blindness. The visual fibres synapse in the lateral geniculate body. Because of the synapse one does not see optic atrophy after lesions of the visual cortex and optic radiation. Superior fibres leave the geniculate body and travel via the optic radiation in the posterior limb of the internal capsule to terminate in the visual cortex. The inferior fibres form a loop (Meyer's loop) around the temporal horn, five centimetres from the tip of the anterior temporal lobe. Hence, the temporal lobe lesions produce incongruous upper quadrantic field defect. The decussation of nasal fibres results in each occipital lobe controlling temporal fibres of the same side and nasal fibres of the opposite side. Fibres from the macula end posteriorly at the tip of the occipital lobe and each fovea projects to both the occipital lobes. Therefore, homonymous hemianopia does not reduce the visual acuity.

Retinal lesions can produce metamorphopsia. On the other hand flashes of light suggest active or irritant lesion of the retina or optic nerve. Lesions of the optic nerve lead to diminution of acuity of vision and to scotomas defined as islands of loss of vision. Scotomas can be positive or negative. Positive scotomas are due to macular lesions and are perceived as grey or black spots in the field of vision. The negative scotomas are due to optic nerve lesions that appear as areas of absent vision in the field. The lesions of retina and optic nerve produce field defects in the ipsilateral eye. Ischaemic optic neuritis generally produces altitudinal field defects. Midline lesions of the chiasm produce binasal loss of field of vision. The binasal field defect could also be due to ischaemic optic neuritis, optic nerve lesions due to nerve hypoplasia, or congenital optic nerve pits, hydrocephalus and basal tumours. True bitemporal field defect is almost always due to chiasmal lesion. Lesions of the optic pathway posterior to the chiasm lead to defects in perception of certain parts of the visual field. The defect in one half of visual field is described as hemianopia. This can be either congruous or incongruous. The anterior retrochiasmal lesion produces incongruous field defect. Anterior occipital cortical lesions produce congruous hemianopia with macular sparing. The extent of visual field loss differs for different colours being maximal for white and minimal for green.

Optic neuritis and papilloedema usually lead to a decrease in the acuity of vision for distant objects. Loss of vision for near objects occurs in ophthalmic conditions. Visual acuity is tested by Snellen's chart. Letters of decreasing size are arranged in rows on the chart with largest letters on the top. The size of the letters is standardised so that a person with normal vision can read the top row of letters at a distance of 60 meters. The next row of letters can be read at 36 meters, the row below it at 12 meters and last row at six meters. The distance between the chart and the patient is 6 meters. Since a person with normal visual acuity can read the smallest letters at a distance of 6 meters, his acuity is expressed as 6/6, whilst person with marked decrease in visual acuity may have acuity of 6/60. If the person in not able to read the chart at all, acuity is then assessed by asking him to count fingers.

At the bedside the field of vision is tested by the "confrontation method". The examiner's vision is taken to be normal and compared to the patient's vision. The examiner sits or stands in front of the patient at a distance of about 3 feet. The patient is asked to cover one eye and the examiner then covers his own eye that is directly opposite to the patient's covered eye. The patient is instructed to keep looking into the examiner's eye. A small object held in the examiner's hand is slowly brought into the field of vision from the periphery. Patient is asked to indicate by the word "yes" or movement of his finger as soon as he perceives the object. Each quadrant is tested individually. If the patient perceives the object at the same time as the examiner his field is said to be normal.

In children and obtunded patients the field of vision is tested by the "menace test". Reflex blinking occurs when a moving object suddenly appears before the eye. To test different quadrants the examiner suddenly brings his hand in from different directions and the presence or absence of blinking is noted.

In parietal lobe lesions, the patient may be unable to perceive objects in one visual field *'visual inattention'* in the presence of a normal visual field. Visual inattention is tested by asking the patient to keep both his eyes open and the examiner stands opposite the patient and puts up different numbers of his fingers of both hands simultaneously in both right and left quadrants. Patient is asked to add up the number of fingers of both hands perceived by him. Patient with visual inattention will not add the fingers perceived in one quadrant as he does not perceive them. The different types of field defects that are commonly seen are listed in Table 2.7

Table 2.7

Different Types Of Visual Field Defects

1.	**Optic nerve**		
	a. Retrobulbar neuritis		Scotomas &loss of acuity of vision
	b. Papilloedema		Concentric narrowing
	c. Glioma and other tumours		
	d. Optic neuropathy due to ischaemia		Altitudinal field defect
2.	**Chiasmal lesions**		
	a. Tumours of pituitary	}	Bitemporal or binasal field defects
	b. Basal tumours	}	
	c. Hydrocephalus	}	
	d. Carotid artery aneurysm	}	
	e. Arachnoiditis- Tuberculous	}	
	f. Tumours in and around chiasma	}	
3.	**Tract lesions**		
	a. Vascular accidents	}	Incongruous hemianopia with
	b. Injuries	}	macular sparing
4.	**Temporal lobe**		
	a. Tumours,abscess, injury	}	Uupper quadrantic hemianopia
5.	**Radiation lesion**		
	a. Vascular accidents	}	Congruous hemianopia
	b. Head injury	}	No macular sparing
5.	**Calcarine fissure lesion**		
	a. Cerebro vascular accidents		Congruous hemianopia with macular sparing
	b. Tumours		

Ophthalmoscopic examination is done with an instrument called the ophthalmoscope and is an essential part of the neurological examination. It allows the physician to view the optic disc or the nerve head, the blood vessels, the retina and the macula. The disc may reveal optic neuritis (papilitis), optic atrophy or papilloedema. In retrobulbar neuritis no changes are discernible on ophthalmoscopic examination. The blood vessels may show arteriosclerosis, arteritis, cholesterol emboli and aneurysms. Retinal examination may show retinitis pigmentosa, retinal detachment or chorioretinitis. Subhyaloid haemorrhage is a preretinal haemorrhage seen in subarachnoid haemorrhage. In lipidosis, a cherry red-spot is seen at macula. The macular flare and star are seen in hypertension, renal disease and with papilitis in neuroretinitis.

Papilloedema may occur due to increased intra-cranial pressure from tumours, blocks in the CSF pathways, hydrocephalus and cerebral oedema. It is also seen in malignant hypertension and in metabolic disorder such as hypercapnia, hyperparathyroidism and sometimes in Guillain-Barre syndrome

Optic neuritis can be of sudden onset or gradual. It could be either mono-ocular or bi-ocular. Retrobulbar neuritis occurs more often in adults and is usually associated with demyelination. Neuritis due to demyelination, infections and vascular lesions usually is of sudden onset. In demyelination, the neuritis is more often retrobulbar as compared to neuritis of the optic nerve head. There is rapid mono-ocular visual loss. Pain and discomfort in and around the eye may precede the visual loss by a day or two, and this generally persists for few days. There is marked impairment of colour vision even when the visual loss is not severe. There is a central scotoma. Involvement of the other eye may occur after few days to few weeks. Prognosis is usually good. More than 80 per cent recover their vision after the first attack. Intravenous methylprednisolone 1 gm daily for three days followed by oral prednisolone is the treatment of choice. In India, approximately 60 % of patients, more females than males, with optic neuritis develop multiple sclerosis on long-term follow up while 70% to 90% of patients with multiple sclerosis develop optic neuritis in the course of their illness.

Parainfectious optic neuritis occurs following measles, mumps, chicken pox, whooping cough and infectious mononucleosis. It is more common in children than adults. It generally occurs 1-3 weeks after the viral fever. It is usually neuroretinitis and involves macula in its course. Headaches, seizures and ataxia may accompany the neuritis.

The toxic neuritis is generally non-painful, bilateral with insidious onset. There is almost always loss of red-green colour vision. One per cent of patients on ethambutol develop optic neuritis after two to seven months of drug ingestion. Prognosis is good. Treatment is stoppage of drug.

Ischaemic optic neuritis could be either anterior or posterior ischaemic optic neuropathy. This could be either segmental or generalised. In anterior ischaemic optic neuropathy, there is usually occlusion of short posterior cilliary arteries. It occurs at the age of 45 -65 years. It can be an isolated event in hypertension. There is usually sudden painless mono-ocular visual loss. There is diffuse or sectorial oedema with splinter shaped haemorrhages. The visual loss is usually altitudinal involving the inferior field. There is also loss of colour vision, but this improves even though the visual acuity may not. Carry out serological studies, lipid profile and exclude diabetes. Serum viscosity, fibrinogen levels and packed cell volume should also be studied. Long-term aspirin is the line of treatment.

Anterior ischaemic optic neuropathy can also occur with giant cell arteritis. The giant cell arteritis involves, superficial temporal, posterior cilliary, ophthalmic and vertebral arteries. The intracranial arteries are spared as they have less elastic tissue. There are headaches, scalp tenderness and claudication of the maxillary muscles. It can be a part of polymyalgia rheumatica syndrome in which there is pain and stiffness of the proximal limb muscles, which is worst in the morning and after exertion. There is associated neck pain, weight loss, anorexia, fever, malaise, night sweats and depression. The arteries are tender, nodular and inflamed. Dissecting aneurysm, aortic incompetence, myocardial infarction, brain stem stroke and renal failure may develop. The ESR and 'C' reactive protein are raised. Prednisolone is the treatment of choice and is continued in maintenance dose till both ESR and 'C' reactive protein normalises.

The causes of optic neuritis are listed in the Table 2.8

Table 2.8

Causes Of Optic Neuropathy

1. Inflammatory	Arachnoiditis Meningitis- Tubercular, Fungal Cryptococcal Syphilis and AIDS, Tabes, Tabo-paresis Inflammation of the orbit and eye Lyme's disease, Cavernous sinus thrombosis
2. Parainfectious	Following measles, mumps, chicken-pox, Infectious mononucleosis, whooping cough
3. Toxic	Ethambutol, Isoniazide, Vigabratin, Amiodarone Chlorpropamide, Clioquinol, Methyl alcohol Heavy metals, Carbon disulphide, Aniline dyes Tobacco, Quinine
3. Deficiency & Metabolic disorders	Vitamin B complex group deficiency Vitamin B12 deficiency Leigh's encephalomyelitis, Mitochondrial cytopathy Diabetes
4. Trauma	Head injuries
5. Vascular	Central retinal artery thrombosis Cavernous sinus thrombosis Anterior ischaemic optic neuropathy Temporal - Giant cell arteritis Aneurysms
6. Compression	Craniostenosis, Optic nerve glioma Meningioma of the olfactory groove Pituitary tumours, Hydrocephalus Paget's disease of bone (Rare in India)
7. **Heredo-familial disorders**	Leber's hereditary optic atrophy Lipidosis, Retinitis pigmentosa Hereditary ataxias - Friedreich's Optic disc drussen, optic disc pits & coloboma Kjer, Behr and Walfran syndromes
8. Demyelination	Multiple sclerosis, Devic's disease Post infectious - Measles, chicken-pox etc. Schilder's disease, Retrobulbar neuritis

When optic neuritis causes swelling of the nerve head, it may be difficult to differentiate from papilloedema. The following points help in the differentiation.

Table 2.9

Differences Between Optic Neuritis And Papilloedema

		Optic neuritis	Papilloedema
1.	**Onset**	Acute, uni\bilateral	Gradual, bilateral
2.	**Vision**	Total loss Central scotoma Good recovery	Gradual diminution Peripheral constriction Partial recovery
3.	**Colour**	Red more affected	All colours equally affected
4.	**Pain**	Present	Absent
5.	**Vessels**	Arteries narrow veins congested	Arteries normal veins congested

Visual evoked potential (VEP), a recent advance in electrophysiology, allows the estimation of the visual evoked response and detects abnormalities in the visual pathway. It has been of great help in the diagnosis of multiple sclerosis. The technique involves the recording of responses from the occipital region following stimulation of one eye with a flickering checkerboard pattern on an illuminated screen. The time taken for the pattern to be recognised by the occipital lobe is compared to standardised norms. A delay in recognition points to a defect along the optic pathway. Normal time is 100 milliseconds.

THE OCULOMOTOR (third), **TROCHLEAR** (fourth) and **ABDUCENT** (sixth) nerves:

THE THIRD OR THE OCULOMOTOR NERVE arises from an elongated nucleus called Edinger-Westphal nucleus, lying beneath the superior colliculus and rostral to the aqueduct of Sylvius in the mid-brain. Fibres for the levator palpebrae superioris arise from the caudal end of unpaired nucleus, which innervates both levator muscles hence, the nuclear lesion causes bilateral ptosis. The cilliary fibres arise at the rostral end. The inferior rectus, inferior oblique, internal rectus and superior rectus are represented in the nucleus in the descending order. The fibres after leaving the nucleus pass through the red nucleus and the substantia nigra. Before emerging at the interpeduncular fossa, the fibres come in direct relationship with the pyramidal tract.

After emergence, in the basal cistern the third nerve lies between the posterior cerebral and superior cerebellar arteries. It then traverses anteriorly along the tentorial edge and enters the cavernous sinus along the lateral wall of the sinus. It enters the orbit through the superior orbital fissure after dividing into two divisions - superior and inferior. The superior branch is situated lateral to the optic nerve. The inferior branch is the larger of the two divisions. The superior branch supplies the superior rectus and levator palpebrae superioris. The inferior division supplies inferior and medial recti and the inferior oblique. The 3rd nerve supplies all the muscles of the eye except the superior oblique and the lateral rectus. It also carries parasympathetic fibres for the constrictor muscle of the pupil. These fibres arise in the Edinger-Westphal nucleus and travel to the cilliary ganglion with the inferior division of the third nerve and reach the cilliary ganglion via the nerve to the inferior oblique. The cilliary ganglion is situated in the muscle cone just behind the globe. Fibres arise from the ganglion and travel with the short cilliary nerves to innervate the sphincter pupillae or the constrictor muscle of the pupil

In a complete third nerve lesion, the affected eye is closed due to ptosis. When the lid is lifted, the eye is deviated outwards and downwards due to unopposed action of the lateral rectus and superior oblique respectively. To test the integrity of the fourth and sixth nerves the examiner asks the patient to move the unaffected eye medially and observes whether the diplopia disappears. The normal downward movement by the superior oblique in the affected eye cannot be tested, as the paralysed medial rectus does not allow adduction of the eye. The secondary action of the superior oblique is observed when the patient tries to look downwards. The affected eye rotates inwards due to the pull by the unaffected superior oblique indicating intact fourth nerve. In a third nerve lesion the pupil is dilated and does not react to light secondary to involvement of the parasympathetic fibres supplying the pupil.

In midbrain lesion in and near the red nucleus gives rise to ipsilateral 3rd nerve palsy with contralateral hemitremors. This is known as Benedikt's syndrome. In Weber's syndrome, there is ipsilateral 3rd nerve palsy with contralateral hemiplegia. In Claude's syndrome described in 1912 there is oculomotor nerve palsy with contralateral ataxia and dysdiadokokinesia with slow rubral tremor. Aneurysms at the junction of posterior communicating artery and internal carotid artery produce acute painful 3rd nerve palsy with involvement of the pupil. The parasympathetic fibres travel superficially in the superior and median part of the nerve receiving the blood supply from pial vessels. In extradural and subdural haematoma due to head injury, compression of the third nerve, by the herniating temporal lobe (uncal herniation) near the tentorial edge, leads to paralysis of the nerve. Initially there is dilatation of pupil with loss of light reflex followed by 3rd nerve palsy. Aneurysm, pituitary apoplexy, meningioma, carotid-cavernous fistula and granulomatous inflammation due to Tolosa-Hunt syndrome involve the third nerve in the cavernous sinus. Tolosa-Hunt syndrome occurs equally in both sexes in the 4th and 6th decades of life. There is usually steady boring pain around the orbit for a week. 3rd, 4th, and 6th nerves in any combinations with 1st division of trigeminal may be affected. Involvement of the optic nerve is unusual. Steroid is the treatment of choice. Diabetes and hypertension spare the pupil as they involve vasa nervorum, which supplies the trunk of the nerve. Ophthalmoplegic migraine can cause reversible 3rd nerve palsy. Lesion of the inferior division of the third nerve in the orbit produces loss of adduction and depression with dilatation of the pupil. Usually trauma and vascular disease are the main cause of involvement of both superior and inferior divisions. In 25% of patients no cause can be found for the 3rd nerve palsy.

Table 2.10

Causes Of Third Nerve Palsy

Intramedullary	Benedict's syndrome, Weber's syndrome and Claude's syndrome.
In Basal cistern	Aneurysm of posterior communicating artery Trans-tentorial herniation due to tumours and extra and subdural haematoma
In Cavernous sinus	Carotid enlargement due to dissection and aneurysm Thrombophlebitis due to mucormycosis & diabetes Tolosa-Hunt syndrome Pituitary apoplexy
In Superior orbital fissure	Inflammation Meningioma
In Orbit	Tumours, Psuedo tumour of the orbit
Muscle	Myasthenia gravis, progressive ocular myopathy, Mitochondrial disease (this is not real 3rd Nerve lesion but is included here for completion)

THE FOURTH OR TROCHLEAR NERVE arises from a nucleus situated below the third nerve nucleus, in the mid-brain ventral to the aqueduct of Sylvius. The fibres curve around the aqueduct of Sylvius and decussate and cross in the anterior medullary vellum at the level of the inferior colliculus. The right nucleus supplies the left superior rectus. The fibres then course backwards to emerge dorsally, inferior to the inferior colliculus. This is the only nerve that emerges from the dorsal aspect of the midbrain. The fibres then course around the cerebral peduncle to pass between posterior cerebral and superior cerebellar arteries. It then comes to lie in the lateral wall of the cavernous sinus. The nerve then enters the orbit through the superior orbital fissure and supplies the superior oblique muscle.

An isolated lesion of the fourth nerve causes weakness of the superior oblique muscle only. When the patient looks straight ahead the affected eye is rotated minimally outwards producing diplopia with the images on top of one another and the false image tilted towards the true image. To avoid the false image the patient tilts his head slightly away from the side of the affected eye. The diplopia is worse when the patient tries to look down as in reading or going down the stairs.

Congenital lesions of the nerve are frequent. Of the acquired causes of the lesion, trauma and vascular lesions are common. However, aneurysms and tumours rarely involve the fourth nerve.

THE SIXTH OR THE ABDUCENT NERVE arises from a nucleus situated in the dorsolateral aspect of mid-pons, inferior to the floor of the fourth ventricle. Fibres of the seventh nerve before exiting, wind round the nucleus of the sixth nerve, which is a matter of clinical relevance. Fibres of the abducent nerve then course downwards and forwards to emerge at the junction of the pons and medulla. It then enters the prepontine basilar cistern. The nerve then has a long course at the base of the brain. It pierces the dura, travels below the petro-sphenoidal ligament, and enters the cavernous sinus. It enters the orbit through superior orbital fissure and supplies the lateral rectus muscle.

In isolated lesion of the sixth nerve, the eye is drawn inwards. To avoid diplopia, the patient may involuntarily close the normal eye giving the impression of ptosis in the unaffected eye. When the affected eye is closed voluntarily, the ptosis in the normal eye disappears. The patient avoids diplopia by turning the head in the direction of the affected eye.

In isolated lesion of the sixth nerve, test hearing and corneal sensation as acoustic neurinoma can frequently cause abducent nerve lesion. Other causes are raised intracranial pressure, trauma, pituitary tumours and meningitis. In Foville's syndrome, the sixth nerve palsy is associated with facial weakness and facial analgesia due to fifth nerve involvement while in Millard-Gubler syndrome there is abducent palsy with contralateral hemiplegia. 'Moebius syndrome' results in bilateral abducent palsy with facial diplegia. Associated abnormalities include atrophy of the anterior part of the tongue, hearing loss, clubfoot and other skeletal abnormalities.

Table 2.11

Opthalmoplegia; Causes And Type Of Lesions

Site of lesion	Cause of lesion	Nerve involved
Nuclear	Brain-stem vascular disease	Any
	Pontine glioma	Any or all
	Multiple sclerosis	Any
	Wernicke's encephalopathy	Commonly third
	Congenital absence	Any
	Degenerative lesions	3rd and 6th
Posterior fossa		
	Meningitis (TB, fungal	
	Bacterial, syphilitic	Commonly 3rd or 6th
		Carcinomatous)
	Nasopharyngeal carcinoma	Any
	Sarcoid	Any
	Guillain-Barre(Miller-Fisher)	All
	Herpes zoster	Any
	Aneurysms	3rd or 6th
	Increased intracranial pressure	6th
	Migraine	Transient any or all
Lesions at petrous tip	Mastoiditis	6th
	Gradenigo's syndrome	6th with 7th 8th and 5th
	Carcinoma naso-pharynx	All
Lesions in the	Thrombosis	6th later 3rd
Cavernous sinus	Intrasellar tumours	3rd
	Aneurysm carotid	3rd or 6th
Lesions at superior	Tumours of orbit	Any or all
Orbital fissure	Inflammatory lesions	Any or all
Orbit	Pseudo tumour	Any or all
Muscle	Myasthenia, mitochondrial myopathy	

When proptosis is associated with the opthalmoplegia, following conditions need to be considered.

Table 2.12

Causes Of Proptosis

PRIMARY NEOPLASM	Rhabdomyosarcoma Optic nerve glioma Neuroblastoma Lacrimal gland tumour
SECONDARY NEOPLASM	Carcinoma Lymphoma Leukaemia
ENDOCRINE DISEASES	Thyrotoxicosis
VASCULAR DISEASES	Congestive cardiac failure Cavernous sinus thrombosis
INFECTIONS	Orbital cellulitis
IDIOPATHIC	Orbital pseudotumour

These three cranial nerves are generally examined together, as they innervate the extraocular muscles, which work in pairs. The medial rectus of one eye works in tandem with the lateral rectus of the other eye producing the horizontal conjugate gaze. The two medial recti work together, which produce convergence. The eye is moved upward by the superior rectus and the inferior oblique, the former working optimally when the eye is adducted by the medial rectus. Similarly downward gaze is brought about by the actions of the inferior rectus and superior oblique. The former functions well when the eye is abducted and the latter when the eye is adducted.

The movement of the eyes is under cortical control. The lateral gaze is under the control of centres located in the frontal and parieto-occipital regions. The frontal lobes control voluntary eye movements in the horizontal gaze. Fibres subserving voluntary horizontal or lateral conjugate gaze arise from area 8 in the middle frontal gyrus. Other areas in the cortex taking part are the prefrontal cortex (area 46), the vestibular cortex, that is the posterior part of superior temporal gyrus and hippocampus, the parietal eye field i.e. the angular gyrus and supra marginal gyrus (areas 39,40) and supplementary eye field area 6. The fibres descend in the anterior limb of the internal capsule to the pons where they decussate. They end in the centre for conjugate gaze now known by the name of para pontine reticular formation (PPRF). This centre also controls the adjacent nucleus of the sixth nerve. Fibres from the sixth nerve travel in the medial longitudinal fasciculus and crosses over to the opposite third nerve nucleus. This allows both eyes to work in conjunction, the right frontal lobe initiating movement to the left and left frontal lobe to the right. (Fig. 2.5).

These movements are rapid, occur in either directions and are known as *saccades.* The saccades are of various types. They can be intentional and triggered internally with a goal or can be intentional visually guided saccades and are carried out for target searching. They can also be memory guided with a visual and vestibular input. The saccades also move the eyes from one target to another and can be visually and/or auditory guided reflex saccades. Spontaneous saccades occur at rest, during other motor activities to scan the environment. Saccadic movements also occur during REM sleep. Antisaccades are movements deliberately made to move the eyes away from a new target. Saccadic eye movements occur in "pulse-step" manner. Pulse is a burst of high frequency activity that precedes eye movement. In case of a left horizontal saccade, the left lateral rectus and right medial rectus receive a pulse of innervation while the left medial and right lateral recti are reciprocally inhibited. The pulse is generated in the Excitatory Burst Neurones (EBN) located in ipsilateral paramedian pontine reticular formation (PPRF) lying rostral to the abducens nucleus. The EBNs are tonically suppressed except just before and during a saccade by *pause cells* which are located in the nucleus raphe interpositus rostral to the abducens nucleus. For initiation of the horizontal gaze, the pause cells receive input from cerebrum, cerebellum and superior colliculus to stop discharging which in turn allows the EBNs to fire. The inhibitory neurones are situated in the medial rostral medulla just caudal to the abducens nucleus. They project across the midline to the opposite abducens nucleus. Once an image is brought to focus at the fovea, smooth slow movements known as slow phases maintain it there. The 'step' holds the eyes in the new position against orbital elastic restoring forces. To maintain the eyes on target, the muscles receive a tonic innervation from a group of neurones, which are thought to be located in the rostral perihypoglossal nuclear complex and the adjacent rostral medial vestibular nucleus. This group of cells is called neural integrator (NI). The cerebellum and PPRF via the positive feedback loop control the gain and thereby maintain the output of the NI. The tracking of a moving object is called smooth pursuit. Pursuit is controlled by parieto-occipital area in close conjunction with the visual cortex.

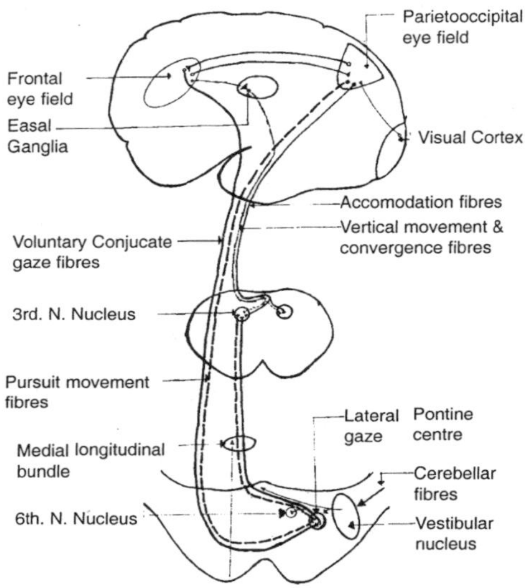

Fig 2.5 Centres and pathways of eye movements

The lesion of the right frontal motor cortex produces the paralysis of the saccade to left and vice versa. On the other hand the lesion in the PPRF produce ipsilateral gaze palsy. However, there is sparing of the vestibulo-ocular reflex and hence, the horizontal gaze with movement of the head will occur.

The Medial Longitudinal Fasciculus (MLF) lesions produce internuclear ophthalmoplegia. In left internuclear ophthalmoplegia the right horizontal gaze is defective leading to loss of adduction of left eye with nystagmoid movements of the right eye. Convergence movements remain intact. There also is vertical nystagmus on movement of the eyes upwards. The horizontal gaze to the left is normal. The causes for MLF lesions are varied. Multiple sclerosis, vascular lesions of the brain stem, tumours in the region of fourth ventricle, paraneoplastic, hydrocephalus and encephalitis can all produce MLF lesion.

When PPRF and MLF are affected on the same side, one and half eye syndrome occurs. The right lesion produces right-sided gaze palsy, and on left horizontal gaze there is defective right eye adduction with normal left eye abduction.

The **VERTICAL GAZE** has a centre in the medial reticular formation (MRF). Some saccades are programmed in PPRF and then relayed to MRF via the MLF. Excitatory burst neurons (EBN) for both upward and downward saccades lie in the rostral interstitial nucleus of the MLF. EBN for upward and downward saccades innervates both ipsilateral and contralateral 3rd and 4th nerve nuclei. The vertical saccades receive bilateral supranuclear innervation from frontal eye fields. The NI (neural integrator - see above) for vertical eye movements is located in the interstitial nucleus of Cajal. They play a role in vertical pursuit movements and eye position. Impairment of upward gaze occurs in Perinand's syndrome. The large pupils, dissociation in light and accommodation reflex, paralysis of convergence and retraction of lid are all associated. There may also be signs due to involvement of other midbrain structures. Usually, the vertical gaze palsies result from tumours of the pineal body and posterior third ventricle, aqueduct stenosis, meningitis, demyelination, mid-brain vascular accidents, arteriovenous malformation, aneurysms and trauma. or neurodegenerative disorders like progressive supra nuclear palsy.

An area in the periaqueductal grey matter controls vergence and the neurones are situated dorsal and dorsolateral to the third nerve nucleus. They project to the medial rectus ipsilaterally. The nucleus reticularis tegmenti pontis (NRTP) is also important. NRTP is contiguous with PPRF and forms a part of feed back loop by relaying visual information to the cerebellum via cerebello-pontine pathways and NRTP functions as vergence integrator. There are vergence tonic cells, burst cells and velocity cells in the periaqueductal grey. The occipito-mesencephalic pathway involved in vergence travels more ventrally in diencephalon and midbrain and hence is less susceptible to compression.

PURSUIT EYE MOVEMENTS: In these movements the eyes move with the moving object and keep the object focussed on the macula or the fovea centralis. This can be termed foveal pursuit. The pursuit movements are also carried out when a target is moving in the visual field and that the slow phase of the optokinetic nystagmus is this type of pursuit. Stimulus from vestibular and ocular pathways can bring about a reflex pursuit movement. The fibres for pursuit movements arise from the area lying anterior to area 19. They also end in the conjugate gaze centre travelling via tectum and tegmentum of the midbrain and pons. Control for pursuit eye movements is located in the ipsilateral parieto-occipital cortex. Additional fibres from the frontal lobes, auditory and visual areas also play a role.

THE PUPILS: The constrictor fibres of the pupils are derived from the parasympathetic system, while the dilator fibres are supplied by the sympathetic nervous system. The size of the pupils at rest depends on the parasympathetic system and intensity of light falling on either eye. The size shape and equality of pupils have to be noted. The direct light reflex is elicited by using a bright light. A poor source of light may fail to elicit the light reflex and lead to false assessment of the patient. On shining a light in the eye, the pupil will constrict briskly. This is the direct light reflex. The indirect light reflex or the consensual light reflex is the simultaneous constriction of the opposite pupil. Accommodation or near reflex is tested by asking the patient to look at his nose and observing the pupils constrict as the patient tries to converge the eyes.

Table 2.13

Pupils

SMALL	LARGE
Old age	Young age
Horner's	Anxiety
Pontine lesion	Atropine
Opiates	Amphetamine overdose
AR pupils	Holmes Adie's syndrome
Pilocarpine	Anoxia, Brain death
	Blind eye
	Carotid aneurysm

THE LIGHT REFLEX: Impulses generated by light falling on the retina are conveyed by the optic nerve to the chiasm. Here nasal fibres cross and both optic tracts now carry the message to the lateral geniculate bodies. Fibres subserving the light reflex are than relayed to the Edinger-Westphal nuclei in the mid-brain. Light falling on one eye causes bilateral excitation of these nuclei; hence there is both a direct and consensual reflex to light. Fibres from these nuclei travel with the third nerve to the orbit (as stated earlier -page 68) lying in the superior aspect of the nerve. The pupillary fibres are located superficially. They finally relay to the cilliary ganglion and supply the constrictor muscle of the iris.

THE ACCOMMODATION OR NEAR REFLEX: Nuclei that control the movements of the medial rectii lie adjacent to the Edinger-Westphal nuclei. When the patient tries to converge he contracts both medial rectii. Impulses from the nuclei of the medial rectii overflow to the Edinger-Westphal nuclei causing the pupil to constrict on convergence.

<u>Lesions of the light reflex pathways</u>: The pupils react normally to light in cortical blindness due to bilateral cortical lesions. Fibres subserving the pupillary light reflex are unaffected as they separate from the visual pathways at the level of the lateral geniculate bodies. In bilateral optic nerve lesions, the pupils are dilated and fixed i.e. they do not react to light. Other causes of bilateral afferent lesions of the pupils are juvenile diabetes, myotonic dystrophy, Perinaud's dorsal midbrain syndrome, pituitary tumours, encephalitis and chronic alcoholism. In unilateral lesion of the optic nerve the pupillary size is unaffected because of the consensual light reflex. When affected eye is stimulated with light neither pupils react while when normal eye is stimulated both pupils react. The accommodation or near reflex is normal. Lesions that compress the midbrain may result in pupils that are fixed and dilated. The Marcus-Gunn pupillary phenomenon or the swinging flash light test is useful in detecting lesions of the afferent arc of the light reflex. When light is shone on the normal eye both pupils constrict briskly. When the light is moved to the affected eye, the pupil paradoxically dilates. This is secondary to a lesion in the afferent pathway, generally the optic nerve. The pupil of the affected eye can constrict consensually

because the efferent pathways are still intact. This pupillary abnormality is seen in retrobulbar neuritis.

Argyll-Robertson pupils(A-R pupils) are secondary to a lesion along the light reflex pathway, at the level of periaqueductal grey matter of the upper midbrain. The pupils are small, irregular, do not react to light, but react to accommodation. There is no pupillary dilatation on instillation of atropine.

Lesions of the third nerve that affect the pupil usually indicate a 'surgical' lesion such as an aneurysm or extra or sub-dural haematoma, whilst lesions that spare the pupil are due to 'medical' causes such as diabetes. Pupillary fibres may be affected in diphtheritic paralysis. Associated palatal palsy may be present.

<u>Lesions of the sympathetic pathway:</u> The sympathetic system originates in nuclei situated in hypothalamus. Fibres descend to the thoracic spinal cord where they synapse. Second order neurones now send their fibres to the superior cervical sympathetic ganglion. Third order neurones send their fibres with the carotid artery to enter the skull. They enter the orbit with the nasocilliary branch of the fifth nerve to innervate the pupils.

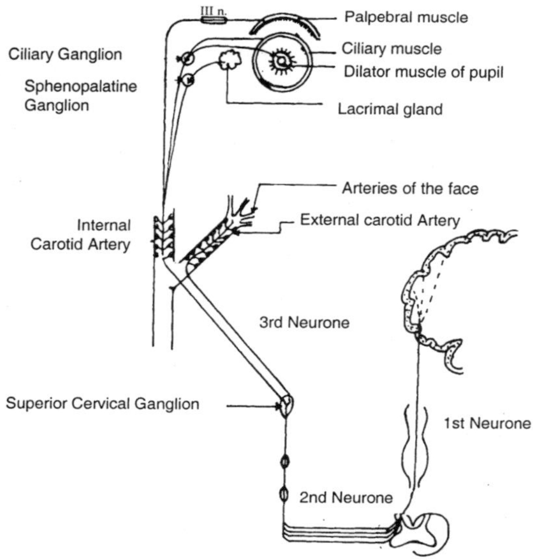

SYMPATHETIC PATHWAY

Sympathetic fibres also innervate the Mueller's muscle, the smooth muscle of the eyelid. A lesion anywhere along this long pathway can result in a Horner's syndrome. The syndrome consists of mild *ptosis* due to involvement of Mueller's muscle, *miosis* due to unopposed action of sphincter pupillae and it dilates slowly. There is *anhidrosis* only if the lesion is below superior cervical ganglion. The eye on the affected side may appear to be shrunken (enophthalmos) due to slight elevation of inferior eyelid because of weakness of inferior tarsal muscle. Finally, the cilio-spinal reflex (dilatation of pupil by giving painful stimuli to the skin of the neck.) may be absent. The pupil reacts normally to light and accommodation. If the lesion is congenital or if of long duration the iris are of different colours.

It is possible to differentiate lesions of the first and second order neurones from the third order neurones by cocaine and hydroxyamphetamine test. When a drop of 4% cocaine is put in either eye, the pupil with Horner's lesion will dilate poorly to cocaine no matter what is the level of lesion. The cocaine test confirms or excludes the presence of the Horner's syndrome. Instillation of 1% hydroxyamphetamine results in dilatation of pupils with lesions of first or second order neurones but not with lesions of third order neurones. Pupillary dilatation depends upon the ability of the third order neurones to produce, transport and store epinephrine. When hydroxyamphetamine is instilled, the pupils dilate because norepinephrine is released. When third order neurones are involved, norepinephrine production and storage is affected. Hence, the pupil does not dilate on instillation of hydroxyamphetamine. The cocaine-hydroxyamphetamine test therefore helps to localise the lesion of the first, second or third order neurones of the sympathetic pathway

Horner's syndrome can result from lesions of the brainstem due to multiple sclerosis, pontine glioma, vascular lesions - lateral medullary syndrome or syringobulbia. Lesions of the cervical spinal cord such as syringomyelia and cranio-vertebral anomalies are other causes of Horner's syndrome. Carcinoma of the apex of the lung - Pancoast's tumour, cervical rib, carotid dissection and aneurysm, malignant or tuberculous lymph nodes, trauma and surgery in the neck cause Horner's syndrome by involvement of the preganglionic cervical sympathetic pathways. The postganglionic lesions causing Horner's syndrome are cluster headaches, nasopharyngeal tumours, otitis media and cavernous sinus lesions. Finally, Horner's syndrome could be congenital or idiopathic. As seen from the list of causes mentioned above, Horner's syndrome per se does not have a localising value.

Adie's pupils are caused by affection of post-ganglionic supply to sphincter pupillae and the cilliary muscles. Mainly it is due to viral infection in young adults. It is unilateral in over 80% of cases. The affected pupil is large and regular. The light reflex is absent. It constricts slowly on accommodation and is tonic with redilatation also being slow. There may be associated autonomic nerve dysfunction and diminution of deep tendon reflexes specially the ankle reflex.

NYSTAGMUS is described at this time as it is generally noted while examining the eye movements, though the lesions that cause the nystagmus are usually located in the vestibular pathways. Nystagmus is a disturbance of ocular posture which is characterised by involuntary, oscillatory, to and fro movements of the eyes. The nystagmus could be either jerky or pendular. It may be horizontal, vertical or rotary. In jerky nystagmus there is a tendency for the laterally deviated eyes to drift slowly to midline, with a fast flicker of movement to the original position. The nystagmus is designated after the direction of the fast component; for instance if the fast component is to the right the nystagmus is called a right nystagmus. However, it is the slow drift of the eyes which is secondary to the pathological lesion, the fast jerky component is the corrective movement undertaken to regain the original position. The nystagmus increases in intensity when one eye is covered.

Fine, jerky nystagmus of moderate frequency seen in extreme lateral gaze is usually a physiological nystagmus. Optokinetic nystagmus is a jerky nystagmus induced by repetitive stimuli moving across the visual field, such as the one induced by watching a train moving along the platform. In this the slow phase is the pursuit movement watching a compartment of the train go by and the fast component is a saccadic movement returning the eyes to the next approaching compartment. The parieto-occipital region controls the slow phase while the frontal lobe controls the fast saccadic phase. Moving a striped drum in front of the eyes also induces it.

'Pendular' nystagmus has equal velocity on both directions. It is seen in ocular lesions with diminished visual activity such as optic atrophy, albinism, congenital cataracts, and total colour blindness. It could also be of central, brainstem or cerebellar in origin. Congenital nystagmus is pendular in type and is present from birth. It tends to convert into jerky nystagmus on lateral gaze. It may be familial, inherited as either sex-linked recessive, affecting males only or may be of autosomal dominant inheritance. The movements can be gross and may be associated with head nodding. The nystagmus disappears on convergence and in sleep. The head nodding disappears over a period of time. This type of nystagmus should be distinguished from other types of pendular nystagmus.

Nystagmus is divided in to three degrees. First degree or minor nystagmus is present only when the eyes are deviated to the extremes of lateral gaze. Second degree nystagmus is apparent with minimal deviation of the eyes and the third degree nystagmus is seen when the eyes are in resting position.

Jerky nystagmus may occur due to lesions anywhere along the vestibular pathways. There is altered input from the vestibular nuclei to the horizontal gaze centre in the PPRF. The slow component of the nystagmus is by the vestibular nuclei, while the fast phase is by fronto-mesencephalic pathway and the brainstem. Chronic lesions of the cochlea such as Meniere's disease and tumours of the vestibular nerve such as acoustic neuroma may not be associated with nystagmus if central compensation has occurred. Nystagmus is marked in acute lesions such as labyrinthitis or neuronitis, till central compensatory mechanisms have been established. As brainstem lesions affect these compensatory mechanisms, nystagmus is always seen with lesions of the brainstem. The nystagmus may be horizontal, vertical or rotary. It is important to differentiate the nystagmus arising from the central lesions from that of the peripheral lesions.

Table 2.14

Central And Peripheral Nystagmus

	CENTRAL	PERIPHERAL
Duration	Short	Prolonged: years
Vertigo	Linked	Dissociated
Direction	Unilateral, horizontal, conjugate	Multidirectional, vertical could be dysconjugate
Effect of loss of fixation	Increased	Not increased

Vertical upbeat nystagmus usually indicates an intrinsic lesion of the brainstem, such as multiple sclerosis, a glioma or an infarct. It also occurs in posterior fossa lesions, Wernicke's encephalopathy or with drug toxicity. The downbeat nystagmus is usually seen with lesions of the cranio-vertebral junction at the level of foramen magnum, such as Arnold-Chiari malformation or syringo-bulbia. It is also seen in Wernicke's encephalopathy, hydrocephalus and drug toxicity.

The left vestibular pathways move the eyes to right. Hence, the eyes will tend to drift towards the left with a lesion on this side. A corrective fast component occurs to the right; therefore the left vestibular lesions produce right nystagmus. To test the intactness of the vestibular pathways caloric test has been devised. In the caloric test 250ml of cold (30 degrees C) and warm water (44 degrees C) is instilled in the ear with a thin catheter attached to a syringe. Instillation of cold water in right ear will induce left nystagmus while hot water will produce right nystagmus. This nystagmus can be recorded electronically and the technique is called electronystagmography.

Cerebellar lesions result in nystagmus towards the diseased side, looking away from the midline, which is due to involvement of the vestibular connections of the cerebellum. Some cases of cerebellar nystagmus require closing the eyes, or examining the patient in a dark room, before the nystagmus is observed.

As stated earlier, in internuclear ophthalmoplegia commonly seen in multiple sclerosis, the lesion is located in the medial longitudinal fasciculus. There is failure of adduction on lateral gaze and nystagmus may be seen in abducting eye. This nystagmus is also known as ataxic nystagmus.

In spasmus nutans, high frequency, small amplitude horizontal nystagmus is seen with nodding of the head. The nystagmus can be unilateral or bilateral and if bilateral, may be asymmetrical. If idiopathic, it disappears by 3 years of age. At times it is due to a glioma of the anterior visual pathways or associated with a porencephalic cyst.

The latent nystagmus occurs due to infantile esotropia leading to dissociated vertical deviation. It becomes apparent on covering one eye and the fast phase of the nystagmus is in the direction of uncovered fixing eye. It disappears when both eyes are open.

Convergence-retraction nystagmus is a jerky nystagmus and is brought about by attempted up-gaze. The fast phase of the nystagmus brings two eyes together as in convergence. It occurs with lesions of the pretectal region, such as pinealoma or brainstem vascular accidents.

In sea-saw nystagmus, one eye elevates and intorts and the other depress and extorts and then the nystagmus reverses direction. It is seen in parasellar tumours, syringo-bulbia and brainstem strokes.

Periodic alternating nystagmus is a jerky nystagmus that rhythmically changes amplitude and direction. It is usually seen in ataxia-telengiectasia or Arnold-Chiari malformation.

Ocular flutter and opsoclonus is a multiplanner conjugate movement of the eyes without compensatory pause, caused by neuroblastoma, viral encephalitis or demyelination. Dancing eyes and dancing feet syndrome is also seen in viral encephalitis.

Ocular bobbing is a rapid, conjugate downward beat of the eyes with slow drift upwards. It is caused by intrinsic pontine lesions or cerebellar lesions, which compress the pons. At times it is seen in metabolic encephalopathy.

Table 2.15

Type Of Nystagmus And Lesions

	TYPE OF NYSTAGMUS	LESION
1.	Rotary	Labirynth
2.	Abducting eye	Medial longitudinal fasciculus
3.	Vertical	Brainstem /cerebellum
	Down beating	CV junction
4.	See saw	Para pituitary lesions
5.	Positional	Utricle
6.	Alternating	Unknown
7.	Pendular	Poor vision
8.	Rebound	Cerebellum
9.	Bruns	C P Angle
10.	Opsoclonus	Brainstem pause neurons

TRIGEMINAL NERVE: (Fifth cranial Nerve). It is a mixed nerve, conveying sensation from the face and providing the motor supply to the muscles of mastication. Sensory fibres from the face terminate in Gasserian ganglion. Second order neurone fibres relay to the brainstem, from where they take diverse courses. Fibres carrying tactile, and discriminatory tactile sensations from the face, course cephalad from the primary sensory nucleus in the pons to the midbrain. Fibres carrying thermal and pain sensations form the descending tract of the trigeminal nerve and end in the elongated nucleus that lies by the side of the tract. The tract and nucleus descend to the first cervical segment of the spinal cord. The fibres are arranged so that fibres carrying sensation from the upper face lie in the lowest part of the tract and those from the lower face lie in the uppermost part of the tract. The mesencephalic nucleus of the fifth nerve receives propioceptive impulses from the muscles of mastication.

The motor fibres originate from the nucleus that lies medial to the large sensory nucleus in the pons. The nerve emerges from the pons as two closely approximated roots, a comparatively small motor root and a larger sensory root. The nerve pierces the dura at the apex of the petrous bone to form the Gasserian ganglion.

The trigeminal nerve has three divisions, the ophthalmic, maxillary and mandibular. The ophthalmic division supplies the conjunctiva, the lacrimal gland, and the skin of the nose, scalp, forehead and the upper eyelid. The maxillary division supplies the skin of the lower eyelid, most of the upper lip, the cheek, temporal area, the nasal mucosa, pharynx, soft palate and tonsils. The mandibular division supplies the lower part of face, the lower lip, the lower teeth and the salivary glands. The motor root travels with the mandibular division to supply the masseter, temporalis and pterygoid muscles.

The ophthalmic division, carries sensations from forehead, temples, scalp meninges and nasal sinuses, the maxillary division from upper jaw, teeth, upper buccal mucosa, tongue and the mandibular division carries sensations from lower jaw and teeth. Trigeminal ganglion lies in Meckel's cave, and contains the cell bodies; the first order neurons for the above- mentioned three divisions of trigeminal nerve. The central projections enter the pons and relay into various nuclei and follow different paths depending upon the modality of sensation they carry. Pain and temperature fibres from ipsilateral face and forehead enter the pons and descend as spinal tract of trigeminus. This tract terminates in the second order neurons, which is spinal nucleus of trigeminus, a long thin nucleus extending down and continuous with substantia gelatinosa of spinal cord. Ophthalmic division fibres terminate in lower part of nuclei (at the level of C1, C2) while mandibular division terminates in the upper part. The second order fibres, arising from spinal nucleus of trigeminus cross to opposite side and ascend to thalamus as trigemino-thalamic tract and then third order fibres project to cortex. Discriminative fine touch relays in principal sensory nucleus in pons and crosses to opposite side to ascend with trigemino-thalamic tract. Proprioceptive fibres from head, subserving the proprioception from mandibular joint and muscles of mastication relay to mesencephalic nucleus and ascend cephalad to thalamus. Important connections are made with motor nucleus of trigeminal nerve, which mediates the stretch reflex of the masticatory muscles and maintains the tension of the bite. Patient is asked to open his mouth slightly. Should not push it wide open. The examiner then places the left forefinger below the lower lip. With a knee hammer he taps on the finger in the downward direction. There may be a slight palpable jerk. This is called 'jaw jerk'. In most of the normal people this is absent.

Facial sensation is checked with a wisp of cotton first. Twisting the cotton wisp to a point and touching the lower and outer portion of the cornea checks the corneal reflex. The patient is asked to look upwards and inwards. If the corneal reflex is present, both the eyes will blink simultaneously. The afferent arc of the corneal reflex is via the ophthalmic division of the fifth and the efferent arc is via the seventh nerve, which supplies the ocularis oculi. If the fifth nerve is involved, there will be no response from either lid when the abnormal side is stimulated, or a normal response from both the lids when the normal side is stimulated. If, on the other hand, the seventh nerve is involved, there is no response on the side of the facial paralysis, irrespective of the side being stimulated.

The pterygoid muscles open the jaw and simultaneously pull it forwards. Weakness of the pterygoids results in deviation of the jaw to the weaker side on opening the mouth. This jaw deviation is best observed by keeping the relative position of the central incisor teeth as a guide, or by keeping one finger in the midline under the chin and asking the patient to open his mouth slowly. Remember the jaw deviates to the side of the lesion. Asking the patient to bite hard and appreciating the contraction of the muscles on palpation tests function of the masseter and temporalis muscles.

TRIGEMINAL NEURALGIA: This extremely painful condition affects one or all three divisions of the trigeminal nerve. The second and third divisions are commonly affected. Women are affected twice as commonly as men. The disease is seen in our country after the age of forty. There is usually no known cause. In a small proportion of cases, it is believed that a vessel - mostly an artery, compresses the root as it comes out of the brainstem. In 25 per cent of patients venous compression is the cause. Associated hypertension is noted in almost 60-70 % of patients.

Pain occurs in paroxysms lasting for one to two minutes. The attacks are described as agonising, the pain being sharp, electric shock-like and lancinating. The patient is free of pain between the attacks. Since facial movement may trigger the attacks, the patient appears very apprehensive and is afraid to move his facial muscles. Speaking, eating, shaving, brushing the teeth or even a blast of air on the face may precipitate attacks. There are often "trigger" points on the face, which, if touched, may set off an attack. The disease generally has a relapsing and remitting course. Each relapse lasts for a longer time, the periods of remissions getting shorter. In trigeminal neuralgia no sensory or motor deficit can be demonstrated on examination of the areas supplied by the trigeminal nerve. The corneal reflex is normal. If a deficit is present, a tumour or vascular malformation should be suspected and appropriate investigation undertaken. Trigeminal neuralgia is also known as "tic douloureux" because muscle twitches accompany the pain during an attack.

Carbamazepine is very effective in controlling the pain. 100 to 200 mg given as a single dose affords relief for a few hours, the same dose being repeated according to the patient's requirements. Gabapentin in a single dose of 300 mg can be tried and again repeated according to patient's requirements. Phenytoin, Valproate and Clonazepam are also known to help relieve the pain. Baclofen 30 - 100 mg in divided doses is also known to help. Amitryptiline 10-75 mg per day helps relieve anxiety and stress. It also helps in relieving pain. If pain proves intractable to medical therapy, alcohol injection of either the peripheral branch such as supra or infra orbital or mental or root or Gasserian ganglion should be considered. Heat coagulation of the root by using radio frequency current has been tried successfully and is the treatment of choice before surgery is contemplated. Surgically, relieving the compression of the root by the loop of an artery near the brainstem is advocated by many neurosurgeons. Prior Magnetic Resonance Imaging (MRI) helps to verify the compression. Approximately 70 -90 per cent do not have recurrence of pain for over ten years, after the operation. Recently, stereotaxic radio surgery of the root with gamma knife has been tried.

Table 2.16

Syndromes Of The Fifth Nerve

Dorsal pons	6th and 7th nerve on the same side	Vascular, tumour
Lateral medulla	Pain and temperature loss contralaterally, ipsilateral VII, Honer's, vertigo, nystagmus	PICA
High central medulla	Onion peel analgesia	Syringobulbia
Lateral central medulla High cervical cord	Balaclava analgesia	Syringomyelia
CP angle	Ipsilateral VII, VIII, nystagmus	Acoustic neuroma, meningioma
Petrous temporal bone	Ipsilateral VI	Middle ear infection, tumour

FACIAL NERVE (Seventh Cranial Nerve): The motor component of the facial nerve together with its sensory-parasympathetic component - the nerve intermedius - emerges from the brainstem in the region of the cerebello-pontine angle. The sensory root carries pain fibres from the external auditory meatus and a small area of the skin between the pinna and the mastoid. The motor root arises from its nucleus situated in the rostro-lateral part of the pons. The nerve in its intra-pontine course winds around the nucleus of the abducens nerve and emerges from the ventral surface of the pons accompanied by nervus intermedius. It lies in close proximity to the eighth nerve as it enters the internal auditory meatus. Within the auditory canal the facial nerve and the nervus intermedius continue in its own canal called the facial canal or the Fallopian canal giving off a branch to the stapedius muscle. The chorda tympani, a branch of the facial nerve carries special visceral afferent fibres arising from bipolar neurones of the geniculate ganglion carrying taste fibres from anterior 2/3rd of the tongue. The central axons of these cells travel with nervus intermedius to end in nucleus solitarius. The peripheral axons separate from the facial nerve before it leaves the facial canal. The chorda tympani then travels with the lingual nerve carrying the taste fibres and parasympathetic fibres to submandibular and sublingual glands. Hence, the geniculate ganglion becomes a significant relay station for efferent and afferent traffic and gives off the superficial petrosal nerve in the Fallopian canal. The facial nerve emerges from the stylomastoid foramen and gives off a branch to supply the posterior belly of the digastric and stylohyoid muscles. The nerve then travels through the parotid gland and divides into a number of branches that supply all the muscles (17 paired muscles) of the face, the frontalis and the platysma. The secreto-motor fibres innervate the lachrymal and salivary glands.

The facial paralysis results in a widening of the palpebral fissure on the affected side, the naso-labial fold is obliterated and there is drooping of the angle of the mouth. However, a very useful sign, detectable even with minimal involvement of the facial nerve, is an absence of blinking on the side of the lesion. As the facial nerve controls the facial musculature testing its function involves testing of the facial movement. The upper division of the nerve supplies the muscles involved in frowning, the intermediate branches supply muscles involved in closing the eyelids and wrinkling the nose, while the inferior branches supply the muscles involved in smiling, laughing, whistling and raising the upper lip. Levator palpebrae superioris the only muscle in the face is supplied by the oculomotor nerve. The patient is asked to frown and wrinkle the forehead, to test the function of the frontalis muscle. Next he/she is asked to close the eyes tightly, burrowing the eyelashes deeply. In a case of facial paralysis, the eye may not close at all, or, if the weakness is minimal, the eyelashes may not be burrowed in deeply. Normally, the eye closure results in the eyeballs rolling upwards, and slightly outwards. In facial palsy, the eyeball is seen to roll up, as the eye cannot be closed due to weakness of orbicularis oculi. This phenomenon is known as "Bell's phenomenon".

The patient is then asked to show the teeth, and say 'eeee'. There is deviation of the angle of the mouth to the normal side, with obliteration of the naso-labial fold on the paralysed side.

In upper motor nenrone lesion involving the face, the frontalis is spared. In upper motor neurone paralysis of the face the emotional movements of the face are less involved than the voluntary movements. While in the lower motor neurone lesions both movements are equally affected. The facial reflexes like the blink and the stapedial reflexes are spared or accentuated in the upper motor neurone lesion while they are suppressed in the lower. Taste and lacrimation are spared in the upper while they are involved in the lower. The table below differentiates between infranuclear and supranuclear lesions of the facial nerve. It also lists the deficits that result from lesions of the facial nerve at various points along its course.

Table 2.17

Differentiation Of Supra And Infra Nuclear Facial Paralysis

SUPRANUCLEAR	INFRANUCLEAR
Frontalis spared	Involved
Less apparent with emotional than voluntary	Both equally affected
Preservation of facial reflexes	Absent
Taste and lacrimation spared	Involved depending on the site of lesion

Table 2.18

Localisation Of Infranuclear Facial Nerve Lesions

a) At stylomastoid foramen and distal to it	Paralysis of facial musculature only
b) In the facial canal before branching of chorda tympani and Gasserian ganglion	Paralysis of facial musculature and loss of taste in anterior 2/3rd tongue
c) In the facial canal before branching of the nerve to stapedius muscle	Paralysis of facial musculature, loss of taste sensation as above and hyperacusis
d) In the posterior fossa	Eighth nerve or other lower cranial nerves simultaneously involved or bilateral facial paralysis
e) Nuclear	Sixth nerve simultaneously involved and other long tract involvement

As mentioned earlier the sensation of taste from anterior 2/3rd of the tongue is carried by the chorda tympani. The taste fibres end in tractus solitarius in the pons. Taste from the posterior 1/3rd of the tongue is carried by the glossopharyngeal nerve to tractus solitarius. From here the relay fibres cross the midline and proceed rostrally with the posterior longitudinal bundle as the gustatory fillet. They end in the hypothalamus. The sensation of taste is tested by first asking the patient to protrude the tongue. Wipe the tongue dry, and then put a drop of sweet or salty substance on the tongue. The patient is then asked to put the tongue back into the mouth and not to swallow till he/she has recognised the taste.

In some instances of facial weakness, there may be a weakness of limb musculature on the same side or the opposite side depending on the level of lesion. These instances will be discussed more fully in the section on the motor system. Bilateral paralysis of the facial muscles is either due to nerve or muscle involvement. In Guillain-Barre syndrome bilateral facial nerve paralysis is at times met with. Patients of facio-scapulo-humeral dystrophy may present with bilateral facial muscle weakness.

Facial nerve is commonly affected in tumours of the cerebello-pontine angle such as acoustic neurinoma, basal meningitis, sarcoidosis, Herpes zoster, otitis, parotitis, the Guillain-Barre' syndrome, trauma, hypertension, diabetes and leukaemia and metastatic lesions of temporal bone.

BELL'S PALSY: The commonest cause of facial palsy is "Bell's palsy" a lesion with no known cause, but where either a viral etiology or demyelination is nevertheless suspected. The suspected virus is Herpes simplex virus. The incidence of Bell's palsy in India is not known however approximately 20 cases/10000 occur in the West. It can occur at any age, though it is uncommon in children and its incidence increases up to the age of forty. There is no predilection for either sex. The onset is usually acute, total paralysis developing in a day or two. Many patients complain of pain behind the ear, for a few days before and after the onset of paralysis. Taste fibres are involved in a small number of patients and hyperacusis occurs when the nerve to stapedius is affected. The normal function of the stapedius is to reduce the amplitude of vibratory excursions of the stapes in oval window. Hyperacusis is an increased acuity of hearing and undue sensitivity to low tones. With unilateral facial paralysis dysarthria occurs. There is pooling of saliva with drooling and while eating the food collects on the side of the lesion. Many patients complain of excessive tearing, due to loss of tone in orbicularis oculi though there is decreased secretion of tears. Unilateral facial weakness is partial in 25 % and total in 75 % of the patients. Eighty per cent of patients recover rapidly and fully. Steroids given early in the illness may hasten the recovery. Sixty to eighty mg of

Prednisolone is given for a week and then tapered rapidly. Physiotherapy helps the patients to deal with the disability but does not speed the recovery. In cases with incomplete or partial recovery, electromyography helps in determining prognosis. The following guidelines are useful to assess prognosis: younger patients with partial paralysis, preservation of taste, good submandibular flow and normal conduction on electromyography will recover fully. If taste and salivation are involved decompression of the nerve in facial canal should be considered.

At times the facial paralysis is recurrent, which is commonly seen with diabetes, sarcoid or leukaemia.

<u>HEMIFACIAL SPASM:</u> Gowers first described hemifacial spasm. He defined it as rapid, irregular clonic twitching of one or more muscles of the face. Muscle frontalis is rarely involved. It usually starts in orbicularis oculi and takes a long time (2-15 years) to spread to other ipsilateral muscles of the face. Stress, psychological upsets and fatigue aggravate it. It may persist in sleep. It can occur after a Bell's palsy and it is due to aberrant regeneration or ephaptic transmission. EMG shows high frequency (approximately 300/sec) rhythmic firing of potentials. Anticonvulsant drugs like Carbamazepine, Hydantoin, Clonazepam and Baclofen have been tried, but usually they are not of great help and ultimately one has to resort to injections of Botulinum toxin in the flickering muscle groups. Botulinum toxin when injected in the affected muscle causes neuro-muscular block by inhibiting the release of acetylcholine at the motor nerve terminal. This leads to diminution of the end plate potential and flaccid paralysis of the affected muscle. Like trigeminal neuralgia, this condition also could be due to an aberrant vascular loop of anterior or posterior inferior cerebellar arteries or their branches, in which case the nerve should be decompressed surgically. Essential blepharospasm - a focal dystonia, is bilateral as compared to facial spasm, which is unilateral.

Facial myokemia, described by Oppenheim, in 1916, consists of continuous ripple like quivering movements of the muscles of the face, which the patient describes as something crawling underneath the skin. It is generally due to intrinsic brain stem lesions such as multiple sclerosis, pontine glioma, basilar invagination or syringobulbia.

Due to aberrant regeneration, fibres for salivary glands end up in lacrimal glands and patients get tearing of the eyes while eating. This phenomenon is known "crocodile tears".

THE ACOUSTIC NERVE (eighth cranial nerve): It consists of two separate divisions carrying the sensation of hearing and balance. The vestibular division arises from the large bipolar cells of the vestibular or Scarpa's ganglion, situated in the distal end of the auditory canal. It travels in the canal with the cochlear division, enters the brain stem behind the facial nerve and ends in four vestibular nuclei. Fibres from these nuclei establish connections with the nuclei of the third, fourth and sixth cranial nerves, the cerebellum, the reticular substance, and centres in the temporal lobes.

The cochlear division of the eighth nerve originates in the bipolar cells of the spiral ganglion in the bony canal of the cochlea and is associated with the hair cells of the auditory receptor organ. The nerve accompanies the vestibular division and enters the brainstem close to the inferior cerebellar peduncle, lying lateral and inferior to the vestibular branch. On entering the brainstem the nerve divides into two branches and ends in two cochlear nuclei. Second order fibres from these nuclei ascend to the auditory centres in the temporal lobes.

The function of the cochlear division is tested clinically by checking the patient's ability to hear sounds of various frequencies including whispered speech in each ear. The Rinne's and Weber's tests help determine whether defective hearing is due to a disease of the inner ear, or of the cochlear nerve. A normal person has better conduction of sound through air than through bone. In Rinne's test, the external auditory canal is blocked with a finger, and then a vibrating tuning fork, which has a frequency of 512C, is placed over the mastoid away from the ear lobule. The patient is asked to indicate when he stops hearing the sound. The tuning fork is now removed from the mastoid and placed in front of the ear. A normal person will still perceive the sound while a patient with middle ear disease will not. This is due to bone conduction of sound better than air conduction in middle ear disease. Also the vibrating tuning fork is heard well in the affected ear, when the fork is placed in the middle of the forehead near the scalp hairline. In this case the Weber's test is said to lateralise to the affected ear. Hearing can be further checked by the use of sophisticated tests such as audiometry and loudness recruitment. The acoustic reflex, tympanometry and electrochochleography are other tests that are used in the investigations of deafness. The auditory evoked potential, tests not only the cochlea but also both the peripheral and central auditory pathway.

Table 2.18

Common Causes Of Sensorineural Deafness

COCHLEAR	Hereditary, viral (rubella, mumps), industrial noise, aminoglycoside antibiotics, Meniere's disease
NEURAL	CP angle tumour, meningitis
BRAINSTEM	Demyelination, infarction, multisystem degeneration

Dysfunction of the vestibular division gives rise to vertigo. Although not a part of routine neurological examination, tests of vestibular function involve alteration of flow of current in the endolymph within the semicircular canals.

CALORIC TESTS: Each ear is tested separately. The patient lies comfortably with the head flexed by 30 degrees so that the horizontal canal lies in the vertical plane. Each ear is irrigated with either 250 ml of cold water at 33 degree Celsius or with hot water at 44 degree Celsius for 40 seconds. The patient is asked to look straight ahead whilst the ear is being irrigated. The patient has a subjective feeling of vertigo and the eyes demonstrate nystagmus to the opposite side if the cold water is used and to the same side if hot water is used. Nystagmus lasts for about two minutes. Electronystagmography is a test, which records nystagmus and may help in differentiating peripheral from central nystagmus.

In Barony's rotation test nystagmus is produced by rapidly rotating a person who is seated in a special chair. Ten revolutions are completed in 20 seconds and the chair is brought to an abrupt standstill. Nystagmus occurs in the direction opposite to the direction of rotation. If there is a unilateral labyrinthine dysfunction, the nystagmus is markedly reduced when the person is rotated in the direction of diseased labyrinth.

The causes of vertigo have already been detailed in chapter one. The causes of deafness are varied and include inherited causes such as Refsum's disease, hereditary sensory neuropathy, deafness associated with spastic paraplegia and facio-scapulo-humeral dystrophy etc. Haemolytic disease of newborn and anoxia at birth affect the auditory pathway and the cochlear nuclei. Head injury commonly produces vertigo and rarely deafness. Viral infections can cause either deafness or vertigo. Drugs that damage the eighth nerve include Quinine, Salicylates, Aminoglycosides, Ethacrynic acid and Frusemide. Tobacco and alcohol have been reported to cause eighth nerve damage. Hypothyroidism and diabetes are some of the metabolic causes whilst vascular lesions of the brain stem, especially a lesion in the anterior inferior cerebellar artery leads to unilateral loss of hearing. Meniere's disease and tumours of the cerebello-pontine angle result in gradual hearing loss

ACOUSTIC NEUROMA: The tumour arises in the vestibular division of the eighth nerve and grows very slowly. Bilateral acoustic neurinomas are almost always seen in patients with neurofibromatosis. Tinnitus is usually the first symptom, followed by gradual loss of hearing. Facial palsy occurs very late in the course of the disease, and is rare despite the close proximity of the facial nerve to the eighth nerve. The tumour compresses the fifth nerve leading to loss of corneal reflex on the affected side early in the course. Numbness over the face may be present, though total loss of sensation is rare. There is generally no pain in the trigeminal distribution. Further tumour growth results in pressure on the brainstem. Ataxia, spasticity, hyperreflexia and an extensor plantar response may be present at this stage. By the time papilloedema has developed, the tumour is fairly large in size. Plain x-rays of the skull reveal widening of the internal auditory meatus. MRI or CAT scan reveals the presence of the tumour early in the course, if suspected. Other investigative procedures include audiometry, electronystagmography, and a study of brainstem auditory evoked responses. Treatment consists of surgical removal of the tumour.
Many drugs are known to produce ototoxicity and following table summarises the common agents.

Table 2.19

Drug Induced Ototoxicity

ANTIBIOTICS	Streptomycin, Gentamycin, Kanamycin, Neomycin, Tobramycin, Vancomycin, Ampicillin, Chloramphenicol, Erythromycin
ANTIMALARIALS	Chloroquine, Quinine
DIURETICS	Frusemide, Bumetanide, Ethacrynic acid
MISCELLAENEOUS	Aspirin, Ibuprofen, Indomethacin, Propranolol, Quinidine

GLOSSOPHARYNGEAL NERVE (Ninth cranial nerve): Though a mixed nerve its motor supply is only to the stylopharyngeus muscle. It also carries taste fibres from the posterior 1/3rd of the tongue. It innervates the parotid glands, the carotid sinus and carotid body. The nerve enters the skull through the jugular foramen. It enters the brainstem in the groove between the medullary olives and inferior cerebellar peduncle. The fibres end in the rostral portion of the nucleus ambiguous in the medulla, in the floor of the fourth ventricle. It has three branches. The first travels to the inferior petrosal glossopharyngeal ganglion and supplies sensory fibres to external ear, middle ear mucosa and Eustachian tube. The second branch is a visceral afferent (parasympathetic) arising from inferior salivatory nucleus and going to parotids, via lesser petrosal nerve to otic ganglion from which post-ganglionic fibres arise and travel via auriculo-temporal nerve in the 3rd division of the trigeminal to supply the parotids. The third branch supplies the carotid sinus and the carotid body.

The afferent arc of the gag reflex is carried via the ninth nerve, the efferent via the vagus (tenth) nerve. When the gag reflex is impaired sensation over the palate and posterior pharyngeal wall has to be tested with a long hatpin. GLOSSOPHARYNGEAL

NEURALGIA is a rare disease that occurs after the age of thirty or forty. The onset is sudden; the attacks are characterised by shooting, stabbing, agonising pain on one side of the palate and pharynx. Swallowing, chewing speaking and coughing readily provokes the attacks. Bradycardia and syncope may accompany the attacks. Sectioning or micro-vascular decompression of the nerve sometimes may control the attacks. Medication is the same as for trigeminal neuralgia.

Apart from schwannoma, singular involvement of the ninth nerve is usually iatrogenic due to surgery in the posterior triangle of the neck or surgery on the carotid artery.

TASTE: The taste is sweet, salty, bitter or sour. Absence of taste is known as ageusia. Total absence rarely ever occurs. Diminished taste sensation is known as hypoageusia and on the other hand increased sensation as hyperageusia. More often distortion of taste occurs which is known as dysgeusia or parageusia. Gustatory receptor cells, which have a limited, life-span and are constantly replaced, are clustered in the taste buds. The buds are located in the papillae situated on the surface of the tongue, back of the mouth and pharynx. The taste fibres from the anterior 2/3rd of the tongue travel via chorda tympani, which joins the facial nerve and is termed nervus intermedius. The nervus intermedius has a station in the geniculate ganglion. Taste fibres from the posterior 1/3rd of the tongue, mouth, soft palate and pharynx travel via the glossopharyngeal to the nodose ganglion. The fibres from these two ganglia enter the brainstem and end in the nucleus of the solitary tract. The central fibres travel upwards via parvocellular division of posterior medial nucleus and then via the posterior limb of the internal capsule end in the frontal operculum and anterior insular cortex. Heavy smoking and drugs such as anti-rheumatic and anti-carcinogenic, Penicillamine, Captopril, Nifedipine and Diltziam affect the taste. Other lesions that affect taste are, xerostomia due to Sjogren's syndrome, radiation, pandysautonomia, primary amyloidosis, high altitudinal sickness, diabetes and vascular and demyelinating diseases affecting the brain stem. In Bell's palsy, at times, the taste from the anterior 2/3rd of the tongue is affected and if impairment persists for 3 weeks, the prognosis for recovery of Bell's palsy is poor.

VAGUS NERVE (Tenth cranial nerve): It is a mixed nerve, arising in the medulla from the nucleus ambiguous and tractus solitarius. It leaves the skull through the jugular foramen with the ninth and eleventh nerves. The auricular branch supplies the concha of the external ear; the pharyngeal branch supplies the levator of the palate, the constrictor of the pharynx, the cricothyroid muscle, and the sensory fibres to the larynx. On the right the recurrent laryngeal nerve arises at the root of the neck and on the left, it arises in the upper thorax. The recurrent laryngeal nerve supplies all the muscles of the larynx except for the cricothyroid. The vagus nerve carries visceral afferent and efferent fibres for all the thoracic and abdominal organs.

Examination of the tenth nerve includes observing palatal movements, the intonation of the speech, and the ability to cough. Bilateral palatal weakness results in a low lying palate, a nasal twang, and nasal regurgitation. Unilateral weakness on the other hand, results in the palate being pulled to the normal side when elevated. It is best observed when the median raphe of the palate is seen to move over to one side instead of going up in the midline. Unilateral vocal cord paralysis leads to hoarseness of the voice, the cord lies immobile in the midline, and the patient is unable to cough normally. A hacking or bovine cough is produced instead.

Lesions that produce ninth and tenth nerve paralysis can be divided into two groups: intramedullary lesions that cause nuclear and supranuclear palsies, and extramedullary lesions that can occur either intra or extra-cranially. Table 2.10 lists the causes of ninth and tenth nerve lesions. Weakness of palate, pharynx and larynx can occur with myasthenia gravis and the patient needs urgent care in such a situation.

Table 2.20

Lesions Causing Nith,Tenth and Eleventh Cranial Nerve Palsies

INTRAMEDULLARY:

LESIONS	UNILATERAL OR BILATERAL	EFFECT
Pontine tumours	Bilateral	Palatal, Pharyngeal Laryngeal palsy
Syringobulbia	Bilateral	As above
Motor Neurone Disease	Bilateral	As above, sensations preserved
Poliomyelitis	Unilateral or bilateral	Can affect any one or all three, sensations preserved
Extramedullary Intracranial		
Cerebello-pontine angle tumours	Unilateral	Gradually progressive palatal, pharyngeal and Laryngeal palsy
Meningitis	Unilateral or bilateral	As above
Guillaine-Barre syndrome (poly-neuritis cranialis)	Bilateral	Palatal, pharyngeal And/or Laryngeal
Diphtheritic neuritis	Unilateral or bilateral	Mainly palate
Extracranial		
Jugular foramen syndromes	Unilateral	9th and 11th or 10 and 11th or 10, 11th and 12th
Neurofibroma, Meningioma, Glomus tumours Recurrent laryngeal palsy-Intra-thoracic tumours Aneurysm of aorta, Left atrial enlargement, Thyroid tumours	Unilateral	Above with Horner's syndrome

ACCESSORY NERVE (Eleventh cranial nerve): It is pure motor nerve consisting of two parts, a medullary and a spinal part. The medullary portion arises from the nucleus ambiguous and the spinal portion from the upper three cervical segments. The spinal portion emerges between the ventral and dorsal roots of the cord, and forms a trunk that ascends through the foramen magnum to join the medullary portion. This common trunk then leaves the skull through the jugular foramen with the ninth and tenth nerves. It supplies the sternomastoid and trapezius muscles. Lesions of the accessory nerve result in wasting and weakness of the sternomastoid and the upper part of the trapezius. The shoulder droops on the side of the paralysed trapezius, the scapula falling away laterally from the thoracic cage, the superior angle being displaced to a greater degree than the inferior angle.

Asking the patient to shrug his shoulders upward against resistance tests power in the trapezius. Asking the patient to turn the head to one side, while the examiner applies resistance to the chin tests the power of the sternomastoid. In cases of bilateral weakness of the sternomastoids, the patient is asked to lift the head off the bed against gravity.

HYPOGLOSSAL NERVE (Twelfth cranial nerve): It is also a pure motor nerve, which supplies the muscles of the tongue – the hypoglossus, styloglossus, genioglossus and geniohyoid muscle. The nerve originates in the hypoglossal nucleus that lies in the posteromedial part of the medulla, beneath the floor of the fourth ventricle. It pierces the dura, enters the hypoglossal canal and on leaving the skull passes vertically downward to the level of the angle of the mandible and reaches the tongue.

Lesions of the hypoglossal nerve lead to atrophy and paralysis of the tongue on the side of the lesion. Fasciculation may be seen when the lesion affects the lower motor neurone. The tongue seems to be full of contracting fibres as it lies in the mouth. On protruding the tongue it deviates to the paralysed side. The patient is unable to press the tongue against the cheek on the affected side.

Carotid dissection and aneurysms, because of its close proximity to the artery affect the nerve. During carotid endarterectomy the nerve may be pulled or traumatised. Attempts at jugular venous puncture can traumatise the nerve iatrogenically. The other causes of twelfth nerve paralysis, are radiation therapy, gunshot wounds, stroke, MS and Guillain-Barre' syndrome. Due to close proximity of the last four cranial nerves, lesions (see Table 2.20) tend to affect them in varying combinations. The presenting symptom remains the same irrespective of the cause. These symptoms include hoarseness of the voice, dysphagia and nasal speech. Bulbar palsy means paralysis of the medullary region and is seen in poliomyelitis or motor neurone disease. Pseudo-bulbar palsy results when cortical fibres to the nuclei of the cranial motor nerves in the bulb are damaged due to any disease.

CHAPTER III MOTOR SYSTEM

In simple terms, the motor system consists of motor neurons and their axons together with the effector organ, the muscle. However, in reality, organization and functions of motor system is a complex process. The motor system consists of the following:

1. **LOWER MOTOR NEURONES:** They comprise of the anterior horn cells of spinal cord (and brainstem cranial nerve nuclei) with their axons, peripheral nerves, which form neuromuscular junctions and the muscles. This is a final common pathway through which we are able to contract our muscles and thus move the joints for locomotion. This final common pathway is influenced by other motor systems described below:
2. **EXTRAPYRAMIDAL SYSTEM:** The basal ganglia with their complex connections.
3. **PYRAMIDAL SYSTEM:** This comprises of corticospinal and cortico-bulbar tracts arising primarily from the motor cortex and controlling the output of the anterior horn cells of spinal cord and the output of cranial nerve nuclei respectively.

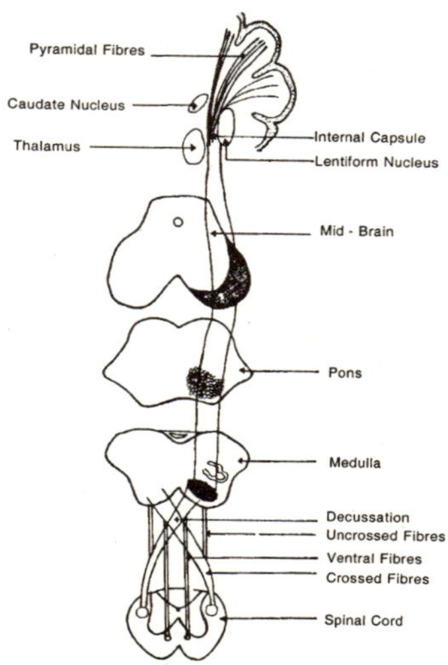

Fig. 3.1 Pyramidal tract and its course

Anterior corticospinal tract terminates in upper thoracic cord and innervates the neurons controlling axial and muscles of the upper extremity while the lateral corticospinal tract continues throughout the spinal cord and innervates the neurons supplying the lower extremity muscles.

4. **CEREBELLAR SYSTEM**: This system coordinates the motor movements

5. **PSYCHOMOTOR LEVEL** : This is the highest level of organization and is concerned with the memory and initiation of motor activity.

The motor system is clinically examined under the following heads:

1. Nutrition
2. Tone
3. Power
4. Involuntary movements

NUTRITION:

Muscle bulk is observed and wasting or hypertrophy is taken into account. Limb circumference is measured at fixed distances from bony points for reproducibility. Wasting can either be generalized as seen in malignancy, thyrotoxicosis, prolonged immobilization or it can be localized to distal (e.g. peripheral neuropathy, distal myopathies, motor neuron disease) or proximal muscles (motor neuron disease, spinal muscular atrophy, muscular dystrophy). Hypertrophy of muscles (especially of the calf muscles) is a feature of some muscular dystrophies like the Duchenne and Becker muscular dystrophy. Rarely, both wasting and hypertrophy is noted in the same muscle group producing 'lump and bump' appearance of the muscle. This is seen in muscular dystrophies like the limb girdle muscular dystrophy and also spinal muscular atrophy (SMA). Along with nutrition of muscles, look for asymmetry of the length of the limbs which may point to congenital maldevelopment, infantile hemiplegia or early life poliomyelitis. Contractures are often seen in muscular dystrophy, SMA and as a sequel of inadequate physiotherapy.

TONE:

Muscle tone is defined as the resistance offered by a resting muscle to passive stretch. It is checked at all muscle joints bilaterally. Tone can be altered in two ways, hypertonia i.e. increase in the muscle tone or hypotonia or flaccidity i.e. decrease in the muscle tone.

Hypertonia is of three types.

1. Spasticity
2. Rigidity
3. Paratonia or Gegenhalten

<u>SPASTICITY:</u> Spasticity is a velocity dependent hypertonia. It is prominent in antigravity musculature, i.e. flexors of upper limb and extensors of lower limb. Spasticity is unidirectional and clasp knife phenomenon may be seen. The clasp knife phenomenon means that after a strong initial resistance the tone suddenly melts away. This is due to Golgi tendon organ reflex. Anatomical basis of the spasticity is the stretch reflex (Figs. 3.2 & 3.3) .

Muscle spindle comprises of intrafusal fibres, which are either the nuclear bag or the nuclear chain fibres. Primary afferents are Group Ia fibres, which innervate both nuclear bag, and chain fibres while Group II secondary afferents innervate only the latter. Axons of alpha and gamma motor neurons, innervating the extra and intrafusal fibres process the efferent arc.

Stretch reflex (or deep tendon reflex) is a monosynpatic reflex, which is the reflex contraction of a muscle in response to being forcibly lengthened. It can be either dynamic (i.e. when the spindle is stretched suddenly e.g. the tendon tapped by hammer) mediated by primary afferents (Ia) of nuclear bag fibres or static (when the spindle is stretched slowly) mediated by secondary afferents (II) of nuclear chain fibres.

The function of gamma efferent system is to maintain the tension in intrafusal fibres thus keeping them duly sensitive to the stretch reflex. More the tension, enhanced will be the reflex. Role of gamma-efferent system becomes clearly evident during locomotion. In locomotion, sustained muscle contraction is needed. Contraction of muscles would lead to shortening of muscle spindle and negative stretch reflex leading to loss of contraction, but gamma-efferent system, by stimulating the intrafusal fibres keeps them in stretched position, thus maintaining the stretch reflex and muscle contraction.

Golgi tendon organ reflex is mediated by an encapsulated sensory receptor located in the tendons. This is a disynaptic reflex with an intervening inhibitory neuron between Ib afferent and the motor neuron. Its function is to monitor the tension in contracting muscles and prevent its excessive rise by inhibiting the alpha motor neuron pool, thus avoiding muscle damage.

Simple reflex arc

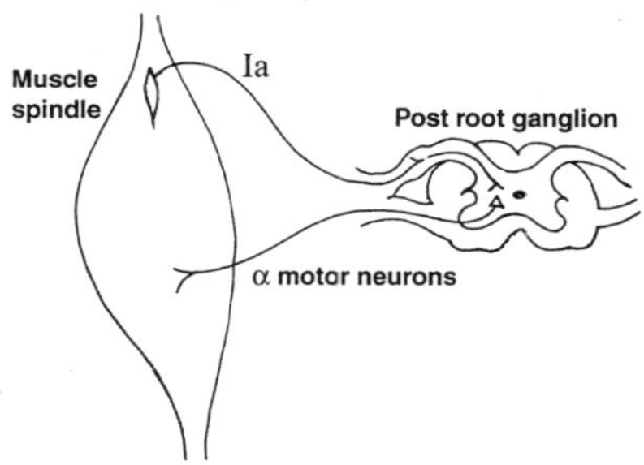

Fig 3.2 Simple reflex arc.

Supra segmental control of the anterior horn cells (α motor neuron)

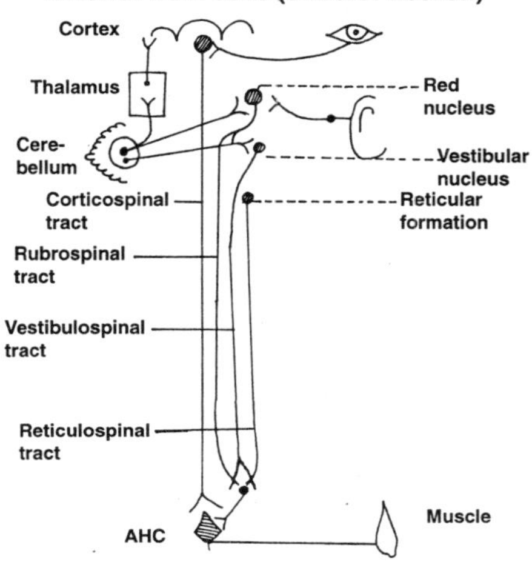

Fig 3.3 Suprasegmental control of stretch reflex

Reciprocal inhibition is a bisynaptic reflex, where the afferent volley via inhibitory interneurons reflexly inhibits motor neurons supplying the antagonistic muscles. This is essential for locomotion.

Flexion withdrawal reflex is a complex polysynaptic protective reflex involving various spinal cord segments where a noxious stimulus produces flexor contraction and inhibition of extension ipsilaterally, thus taking the limb away from the noxious stimuli. This is under inhibitory control of dorsal reticulo-spinal tracts.

Crossed extensor reflex is often associated with flexion withdrawal reflex, involving the extension of contralateral limbs.

RIGIDITY: Rigidity is hypertonia characterized by uniform resistance throughout the movement (i.e. lead pipe) and unlike spasticity, is bi-directional, being equal in both flexor and extensor groups of muscles. Cogwheeling is an abnormal ratchet like sensation associated with rigidity due to the presence of clinical or sub-clinical tremors.

GEGENHALTEN (Paratonia) is a type of hypertonia noted in extensive, bilateral damage to mesial cortex and superior convexity of frontal lobes (Premotor areas). In such patients, attempt to move a joint by the examiner is proportionally resisted by the patient as if he is opposing the movement.

HYPOTONIA (or flaccidity) is a feature of lower motor neuron lesions like the diseases of anterior horn cells, neuropathies and myopathies. In hypotonia, muscles feel flabby and the limb is flail. Joints can be moved to wider range like that of a rag-doll. A child or infant may acquire a frog-leg position. Besides the lower motor neurone conditions mentioned above, the tone may rarely decrease in other conditions given below.

1. Cerebellar Lesions: Pendular jerks may be demonstrated, if the reflexes are intact.
2. Acute Upper Motor Neurone Lesions: During the stage of shock hypotonia may be seen in the first few days of the ictus.
3. Extrapyramidal Disorders: Hypotonia is uncommon in extrapyramidal disorders but may sometimes be seen in cases of chorea.

POWER :

Power is tested by active contraction of muscles / muscle groups. It is graded as per Medical Research Council scoring system, as follows:

5 = Full power
4 = Can over come moderate resistance against gravity
3 = Can move against gravity but not against resistance
2 = Cannot move against gravity
1 = Flicker of movement
0 = No movement at all

Be sure as to which muscle/ muscle group is being tested. Right position of the limb is obtained for that muscle to act alone. Rule out any painful condition, which can limit the patient's cooperation. Power of muscles should be assessed as per the constitution and age of both the patient and the examiner.

TYPES OF MUSCLE WEAKNESS :

Muscle weakness is seen in both the upper and the lower motor neurone conditions. The pattern of weakness, evolution of deficit and the associated neurological signs help the examiner to decide the site of lesion. Weakness should be differentiated from fatigue. In fatigue, the first contraction is strong. Generalized fatigue is encountered in many clinical situations but fatigue of focal areas is seen in myasthenia gravis.

MYASTHENIA GRAVIS

Myasthenia gravis is a neuromuscular transmission defect. In this condition, the muscular weakness fluctuates (diurnally or even hour to hour), increasing as muscle is exercised and then improves as it is rested for some time. Myasthenics are better in cold climates. Initially, weakness is evident in extraocular muscles. Later face, tongue, pharynx and limb muscles are affected. The diagnosis is confirmed by intravenous injection of edrophonium chloride (Tensilon) showing reversal of weakness. Myasthenia gravis is the commonest disorder of the neuro-muscular junction seen in clinical practice and is known worldwide. The disease is seen in both sexes and at almost all ages, though the peak occurrence is around the second and third decades. There is preponderance of young females and elderly males.

Clinical features: The most important feature of myasthenia is easy fatiguability of muscle that is made worse on exercise and relieved by rest. Patients are unable to perform sustained activity. Rest restores the strength. The symptoms have a diurnal variation, with the patient feeling worse in the evening. The muscles supplied by the cranial nerves are most often involved, with resultant ptosis, diplopia opthalmoplegia, dysphagia and dysphonia. The disease then involves the proximal limb muscles. Rarely, weakness appears in the limbs before it appears in the cranial muscles. Muscle involvement is usually asymmetric with muscles of the neck, shoulder girdle and the flexors of the hip being more frequently involved than the muscles of the trunk and legs. Drooping of the eyelids is the commonest symptom. The patient is asked to look upwards and ptosis develops on persistent gaze upwards. The disease begins insidiously but may present acutely after severe emotional stress. Myasthenic patients feel better in the cold weather compared to warmer climates. Exposure to bright sunlight affects the patient adversely. Demonstration of fatigue is perhaps the most important clinical sign for the diagnosis of myasthenia gravis. In very long-standing, non-responding patients, a myopathy may develop. Depending upon the clinical evolution, myasthenia can be classified.

Clinical classification of myasthenia gravis

- Congenital
- Neonatal
- Adult
  - Ocular
  - Mild generalized
  - Moderate generalized
  - Acute fulminant may present in crisis, thymoma more common
  - Severe – similar to acute fulminant but occurring few years after mild or moderate.

Aetiology and pathogenesis:

Myasthenia gravis is an immune mediated disease. Hence it can be seen to be associated with other immunological conditions as mentioned below.

Table 3.1

Diseases Associated With Myasthenia Gravis

Thymic hyperplasia, thymoma	Hyper, hypothyroidism, thyroiditis
Rheumatoid arthritis	Systemic lupus erythematosus
Haemolytic anaemia	Pernicious anaemia
Red cell aplasia	Ideopathic thrombocytopenic purpura
Vitiligo	Pemphigus
Multiple sclerosis	Sarcoidosis
Ulcerative colitis	Leukaemia, lymphoma

It is believed that antibodies develop against the myoid cell elements present in the thymus and these antibodies are directed against the acetylcholine receptors. They bind to the sub units of the receptor and thus disable its function. Hence, acetylcholine released from the nerve terminals cannot make contact with the receptor and hence muscle membrane potential does not change. This results in failure of the neuromuscular transmission. There is a very rapid turnover of the acetylcholine receptors and the number of healthy receptors is constantly changing. Hence the symptoms are constantly fluctuating.

Laboratory Investigations:

Laboratory investigations in myasthenia are mainly supportive. In order to demonstrate reversibility of the weakness of the muscles, the Prostigmine or Tensilon test, can be done by the bedside. The acetylcholine receptor antibodies may be elevated in majority of patients with generalized disease and to a lesser extent, in patients with ocular symptoms. Very high levels are associated with thymoma. Normal level of antibody does not negate the diagnosis of myasthenia. A CT scan of the chest should be done in all patients to evaluate thymus. High-resolution scan is preferred. Electrophysiology is very useful in the diagnosis. Repetitive stimulation at the rate of 3/second shows reduction of the compound muscle action potential, called the decremental response. This response is highly suggestive of myasthenia gravis but can also be seen in a variety of neuromuscular disorders and clinical correlation is essential. Single fibre EMG is now an established test for the diagnosis of myasthenia. Further tests like muscle biopsy and specialized studies of the neuromuscular junction are mainly of research interest. It is important for the clinician to remember the most valuable aid to the diagnosis is the history and the demonstration of clinical fatiguability.

Treatment : Initially, the patients are started on choline esterase inhibitor agents like Neostigmine or Pyridostigmine. The dose needs to be titrated for individual patient and fluctuates from day to day. The side effects like excessive salivation, gut hypermotility and chest secretions can be limiting factors in building up the dose. This effect can be prevented by Atropine. As the basis of the disease is immunological, immunomodulation is a logical mode of management. This helps to induce remission. Corticosteroids are the most widely used agents. The dose could either be gradually increased, or therapy can also be carefully begun with 1-2 mg per Kg doses. The choice depends upon the severity of the disease and also the indoor or outdoor setting of therapy. In the initial periods after institution of therapy, the neurological status can get worse and it is preferable to have the patient under close indoor supervision. As the condition stabilizes and improves, the doses can be gradually tapered. In a proportion of patients, steroids can be tapered off, while others need maintenance doses. Those patients who do not tolerate steroids need to be given other immunomodulants like Azathioprine. Intravenous Immunoglobulins are also useful to bring about remission of the disease. Thymectomy is a must when the patient has a thymoma. In others, it is generally believed that removing the thymus leads to a favourable response, over a period of months and hence may be advised in younger patients. The role of thymectomy in patients having generalized myasthenia with normal antibodies to acetylcholine receptor and in patients with ocular myasthenia is less certain.

Myasthenics may encounter sudden deterioration of muscle power, the crisis. Crisis is generally precipitated by stress and infection. Such patients need intensive care. Airway, respiration and swallowing function needs to be closely monitored and supported. Injectable choline esterase inhibitors need to be used and titration of each individual dose is necessary. The precipitating factor needs to be dealt with. Plasmapharesis is the treatment of choice in crisis. Rarely, the crisis may be due to over use of the cholinergic medication. This needs to be kept in mind when planning the therapy. Over all, the course of myasthenia, in the modern times is favourable and patients can look forward to a useful life.

Hysterical weakness is usually seen in young females who want to seek attention or plan other gains. This weakness does not conform to a known neurological pattern and improves with encouragement. There is marked disparity between the power grade and movement performed by the patient. Often there is a sudden let go while testing power. Similarly, the hysterical gait is a very bizarre gait that does not resemble any specific gaits described in the book. The abnormality increases when the patient is aware that he is being watched.

FASCICULATION: The number of muscle fibres innervated by a single motor neuron is called a fasciculus or motor unit. Fasciculation are fine, rapid, flickering movements. They are visibly noted underneath the skin, are spontaneous (or induced by gentle tap on skin, exercise, cold and cholinergic drugs) contractions of muscle fibres belonging to a single motor unit. Fasciculations can be heard through the stethoscope, on its application to the belly of the muscle. Physiologically, the site of origin of fasciculation appears to be multifocal and the abnormal excitability can arise from distal portion of the axon to the anterior horn cell. Clinically, most frequently, diseases of anterior horn cells (MND, SMA), less frequently radiculopathies and rarely peripheral neuropathies give rise to fasciculations. They can occur in healthy individuals too ('Benign fasciculation'). In this instance, the fasciculations are not associated with any other deficit of the lower motor neurone. Fasciculatory tremors or polyminimyoclonus are fasciculations of small muscles of fingers seen in a variety of conditions.

INVOLUNTARY MOVEMENTS: Observe the patient at rest then ask him to raise the arms with outstretched hands in front of him and hold the position with closed eyes. Further ask him to touch his nose with his eyes open. Finally, ask him to stand up and walk. Most of the disorders of movement will be evident during above - mentioned examination. Following features should be noted about the movement disorder.

Which parts of the body are affected?

Judge the frequency of the movement.
Does it occur predominantly at rest or during action?
Is there any aggravation when the patient tries to touch his nose, which indicates intentional component?
Is there any change during the eye closure?
Does it remain persistent in sleep?
Chorea is involuntary, purposeless, non-stereotyped, rapid, mainly distal movement. Tremors are rhythmic movements due to altered contraction of agonists and antagonists and are of three different types.

1. Rest tremors: Parkinson's disease
2. Intention tremors: Cerebellar disorders
3. Postural tremors: Essential tremors

Table 3.2

Tremor Characteristics

	Rest tremor	Postural tremor	Action tremor
Parkinson's disease	+++	+	-
Essential tremor	------	+++	+
Cerebellar tremor	------	+	+++
Rubral tremor	------	+++	+++++
Physiologic, thyrotoxic, anxiety	------	++	-----

Hemiballismus is a violent flinging movement of the limbs due to lesions in contra lateral subthalamic nucleus. The lesion is usually vascular in origin. Athetosis is a slow writhing movement of extremities. Pseudo athetoid movement (movements that simulate the true athetosis) is an important physical sign that is associated with prominent loss of postural sensibility. It is elicited by asking the patient to raise both hands in front of him and close the eyes. Dystonia is a slow sustained abnormal movement, which can be focal or generalized. Primary dystonia is a neurodegenerative condition, which can have onset either in childhood (e.g. idiopathic torsion dystonia) or during adulthood (e.g. spasmodic torticollis;

writers cramp etc). Wilson's disease must be excluded in any young patient with involuntary movements since it is treatable. Myoclonic jerks are sudden shock- like contractions of a muscle or a group of muscles, which occur singly or two three times in rapid succession. Focal seizures affect one part of the body, without loss of consciousness Asterixis or flapping tremors are noted in metabolic encephalopathies. For further details of common involuntary movements, please see Chapter II.

LESIONS OF UPPER AND LOWER MOTOR NEURONE

Lesions of the descending corticospinal tract of pyramidal system are termed as Upper Motor Neurone (UMN) lesions while the Lower Motor Neurone (LMN) lesions comprise of diseases of the anterior horn cells, roots, peripheral nerves, neuromuscular junction and muscles. It is possible to clinically differentiate these two broad categories of lesions.

In the upper motor neurone lesions, paralysis is generalized rather than focal. It involves either the whole extremity or specific movements of a limb rather than specific muscles. Often, extensors and abductors of upper limbs and flexors of lower limbs are predominantly involved in UMN lesions. In LMN lesions, weakness is focal and commonly affects specific muscles. Muscle tone may initially be decreased in acute corticospinal lesions (shock stage) but with in weeks, the limb becomes spastic. Flaccidity is a feature of lower motor neurone lesions. Wasting is very prominent and severe in LMN lesions especially of anterior horn cells. As much as 70-80% of muscle bulk may be lost in initial 3 months. In UMN lesions wasting is late and limited to disuse atrophy. Fasciculation are seen in LMN lesions and are not a feature of UMN lesions. Deep tendon reflexes may be initially absent in acute UMN lesions (shock stage) but become hyperactive later and may even show clonus. This is associated with the extensor plantar response, the Babinski's sign. In LMN lesions, stretch reflexes are sluggish to absent, in proportion to the severity of weakness. Trophic changes are at times seen in LMN lesions.

Table 3.3.

Differences Between The Upper And Lower Motor Neurone Lesions.

	UMN	LMN
Muscle bulk	Normal	Wasting
Fasciculations	Absent	Present
Muscle tone	Spastic Widespread paresis (Flexors in LL, Extensor in UL) Characteristic distribution of hemiparesis	Flaccid Focal paresis Specific muscles may be involved
Superficial reflexes	Absent	Present
Deep tendon reflexes	Hyperactive	Sluggish to absent
Babinski sign	Extensor	Flexor

MOTOR NEURONE DISEASE (MND)

Motor neurone disease is a progressive disease affecting the motor system. The disease is seen in both sexes and mainly affects individuals above 50 years of age. Cases are known to occur at much younger ages, but at a much lesser frequency. The disease is usually sporadic, and familial occurrence, though definite, is uncommon in clinical practice.

CLINICAL FEATURES: Both parts of the motor system, the upper and the lower motor neurones can be affected. The combination of upper and lower motor neurone affectation is the most common, but infrequently, only the lower or the upper motor neurones may be degenerated. Thus, depending upon which part of the motor system is bearing the brunt of the disease, following clinical types can be identified.

1. Amyotrophic lateral sclerosis: This perhaps is the commonest form of motor neurone disease. Initially, the small muscles of one hand are usually involved, with gradually progressive weakness and wasting of the muscles noted by the patient. Initial difficulty is in performing tasks like opening the lid of a bottle.

Fasciculation may be seen in the affected areas by the patients themselves and their relatives. The weakness and loss of bulk relentlessly progresses to affect more areas of the body in an asymmetric manner and becomes widespread. The neurological examination reveals widespread lower motor neurone signs along with upper motor neurone signs. Therefore, one may see very brisk reflexes in a wasted and weak area. Fasciculation are seen in many segments and their widespread nature is very relevant to the process of clinical diagnosis of motor neurone disease. Even though the upper motor neurones are involved, the superficial reflexes like the abdominal reflexes tend to be normal or brisk producing a dancing umbilicus sign and the plantar response, the Babinski's reflex may not be extensor till late in the illness. In this respect, the pyramidal tract manifestations in this disease are rather different from that of demyelinating diseases like multiple sclerosis wherein the early manifestations may be loss of superficial reflexes, extensor plantar and urinary retention.

When the process of degeneration affects the cranial nerve nuclei and the corticobulbar tracts, the result is a combination of bulbar and pseudobulbar palsy. This development is important for the management decisions.

2. Progressive muscular atrophy: In this condition, only the lower motor neurones are affected and hence the patients present with progressive wasting and weakness of multiple body segments with fasciculation. Since there are no upper motor neurone signs in such patients, the distinction from peripheral neuropathies and inherited anterior horn cell diseases like the spinal muscular atrophy is relevant.

3. Primary lateral sclerosis: This is the least common presentation of motor neurone disease. Here, only the upper motor neurones degenerate and hence result in spasticity, hyperreflexia and extensor plantar responses. In a proportion of such patients, subclinical lower motor neurone involvement may be present and electrophysiology may be required to document it. When indeed, only the upper motor neurone signs are present, a differential diagnosis of hereditary spastic paraplegia and other familial diseases needs to be considered.

The course of motor neurone disease is relentlessly progressive. The speed of deterioration may vary in different individuals but the disease takes its toll within 2-5 years. The development of pseudobulbar state and respiratory muscle weakness signifies advanced stages of the condition. Death is usually related to respiratory and bulbar dysfunction.

UNCOMMON PATTERNS IN MND :

1. Guam MND. A combination of motor neurone disease, dementia and parkinsonian features is seen.
2. Madras MND: The onset is at a younger age around 10 to 30 years. The progress is slow. There is absence of family history. The eighth nerve may be affected. The distal muscles of the upper limbs and the lower limbs are inolved. Foot drop is usually present. The paralysis is asymmetric and facial and bulbar musculature may be involved. The tendon reflexes may be normal or brisk, with extensor plantar responses. Low fasting citrate and elevated pyruvate levels in the serum are reported.
3. MND and dementia may occur in the prion diseases like the Crutzfieldt-Jacob disease.
4. Familial MNDs have been described. The ALS gene in such cases maps to the chromosome 21 and codes for superoxide dysmutase. The familial form is very similar in the clinical course to the sporadic form.
5. Monomelic amyotrophy: Involvement of a single limb either the upper or lower (mostly upper) with weakness and wasting has been described in Asian countries and is labelled as monomelic amyotrophy. It presents around 2nd or 3rd decade and is sporadic. Stiffness and cramps may develop on exposure to cold. Hyperhydrosis may be present. Though forearm and hand muscles are affected, the brachioradialis may be spared. There may be presence of irregular, jerky tremors of the fingers (polyminimyoclonus). Tendon reflexes are depressed and the plantar responses are flexors. The disease involves the anterior horn cells. It can over years involve the second limb or become generalised. Contractures may develop late, the course is benign.
6. Post-polio paralysis behaves more like Spinal muscular atrophy (SMA) and can be diagnosed by obtaining the history of paralytic

polio in childhood and examination shows asymmetry of muscle affection. Initially, the severely affected muscle becomes further weak and the improved activity is lost. The weakness then progresses and becomes generalised. Fatiguability is also noted. Tendon jerks are lost and fasciculations are not comnonly seen.

AETIOLOGY: In spite of efforts, the aetiology of MND is still elusive. Familial case studies have given the link to chromosome 21 and superoxide dysmutase, but whether similar mechanisms are operating in the sporadic cases, which form the bulk of the cases of MND is not clear. The clusters of patients seen in the island of Guam and the other islands on the Western Pacific region suggest an environmental factor in the development of MND but neither the study of the environment nor the genetic studies like HLA studies have given any clear answers. Premature ageing has been a popular theory to explain the untimely decay of the anterior horn cells and the pyramidal cells, but the factors that may be hastening this ageing are far from clear. The similarity of progressive muscular atrophy to motor toxic neuropathies has lead to extensive search for a toxic factor, again, in vain. Recently, a toxin from the plant Cycas circenalis has been shown to result in features like MND in experimental animal models. Viruses have also been popular culprits. The natural existence of polio and polio-like illness of the anterior horn cells makes it an attractive theory. However, to date, no virus has been causally associated with MND. Hexasaminidase A deficiency also produces a disease very much like the MND.

INVESTIGATIONS : The most important investigation is the EMG-NCV study. This establishes the site of lesion to be at the anterior horn cells and also establishes the widespread nature of the process. Hence it is important to tailor the study to suit each patient, ensuring that multiple segments are tested. In the early stages, the anterior horn cell involvement is restricted to few segments and then imaging of the spinal cord or brain may have to be undertaken. Investigations like serum calcium estimation and serum protein electrophoresis are relevant to atypical cases of secondary motor neurone disease.

TREATMENT : As the cause of MND is not clear, it is obvious that therapy is not at hand. In fact, a consultation with a patient of motor neurone disease can be very difficult when it comes to the therapy and needs to be handled tactfully. It is better to slowly introduce the diagnosis and the associated reduction in quality and duration of survival. Multiple interviews with patients and relatives may be necessary. The clinician's best stand perhaps is of an informed friend and guide. The symptoms will need to be treated on their own merit. Stiffness and cramps may respond to anti spasticity agents like Baclofen or Tizanidine. Swallowing and breathing difficulty is of particular importance. If the patient coughs or chokes on food, a nasogastric tube has to be inserted. For prolonged durations, percutaneous feeding gastrostomy can be performed. This is not unsightly like the nasogastric tube as it hides in patient's clothing. Ventilation also needs careful monitoring and support may be required. Chest physiotherapy and deep breathing exercises are important in maintaining the capacity of the respiratory system at its best. Respiratory infections should be identified and treated rapidly as they result in rapid deterioration of the patient's overall condition. Pharmacotherapeutic agents like Riluzole, Glutathione, thyrotrophic releasing hormone, nerve growth factor etc. have been used but without much clinical success. Patients usually succumb to respiratory infection.

HEMIPLEGIA: Hemiplegia means weakness of an arm and the leg on the same side. In general, focal structural lesions rather than diffuse or systemic lesions cause hemiplegia. The gait in hemiplegia is known as circumducting gait because the paralysed lower extremity has dominant extensor tone with inability to flex the knee, and hence while walking the lower extremity makes an outer semicircle as it progresses forward. Anatomical localisation of hemiplegia depends upon the distribution of motor and associated non-motor deficits like sensory, language and cranial nerve dysfunctions.

CORTICAL LESIONS that lead to hemiplegia are usually due to massive middle cerebral artery (MCA) territory infarcts. Cortical lesions producing hemiplegia have to be large because of the 'homunculus' (body representation) in cortex, which requires the lesion to be fairly extensive to result in hemiplegia. If dominant lobe is involved, aphasia, and apraxia are associated. On the other hand, hemineglect is associated when the non-dominant lobe is affected. In cortical lesions without motor deficit, hemisenosry defect due to involvement of sensory cortex and pathways and hemianopia due to lesion in the optic radiation, are seen.

SUBCORTICAL LESIONS are usually due to lacunar strokes in corona radiata, internal capsule and basal ganglia. Lesions in posterior limb of internal capsule, usually lead to a pure motor stroke with almost equal involvement of arm and leg without cortical dysfunction (aphasia, apraxia or hemineglect). Hemisensory loss and homonymous hemianopia may be associated.

THALAMIC LESIONS cause contralateral sensory impairment and amnesia. Thalamic pains may dominate the resulting syndrome.

BRAIN STEM LESIONS produce characteristic findings of hemiplegia with cranial nerve deficits on the opposite side and loss of sensory modalities on the same side as hemplegia. Various syndromes have been described of which common ones are mentioned below.

1. Weber's syndrome: With hemiplegia ipsilateral IIIrd nerve is involved.
2. Benedict's syndrome: A coarse tremor in the arm on the side of lesion due to involvement of the red nucleus associated with contralateral hemiplegia
3. Millard Gubler syndrome: Ipsilateral VIth and VIIth nerve involvement with contralateral hemiplegia.

Lacunar strokes, that is, small ischaemic lesions, often produce following patterns of neurological deficit:

1. Pure motor paresis
2. Pure sensory hemidefect
3. Dysarthria-clumsy hand syndrome
4. Ataxic hemiparesis
5. Hemichorea-hemiballismus

The following distinctive features diagnose hemiplegia due to malingering or conversion reaction.

- Improvement in power with encouragement
- Fluctuating power
- Give-way weakness
- Hoover's sign is demonstrated by asking the patient to lie supine and the examiner's palm is kept under both the heels. In right hemiplegia as the right limb is paralysed, the examiner would feel the pressure of the left normal heel. The absence of the pressure suggests functional hemiplegia
- Presence of gain
- Absence of associated reflex or sensory changes.

Hemiplegia is often the result of a vascular disease of the brain described in common parlance as a stroke.

Table 3.4

The Common Aetiologies Of Stroke:

	Embolism	Thrombosis	Haemorrhage
Onset/progress Deficit at onset	Acute/maximum	Acute/progresses over hours	Acute/Progresses over short duration
Headaches	+	-	+++
Seizures	++	+\-	+
TIA	-	+++	-
Cause.	Cardiogenic\arterial	Atherosclerosis	Hypertension

SPINAL CORD

ANATOMY

Spinal cord is elongated cylindrical mass of nerve tissue occupying the upper 2/3rd of vertebral canal. During foetal development it extends throughout the vertebral column but since the growth of bony vertebrae is faster, the cord tends to extend up to the level of L_3 vertebra at birth and subsequently comes to lie in its adult position - lower border of L_1. Total 31 pairs of spinal nerves exit from their respective cord segments (8 cervical, 12 thoracic, 5 lumbar, 5 Sacral and 1 coccygeal). Due to different rates of growth of bony vertebrae and spinal cord the relationship of spinal segments and bony vertebra merits a special mention

In cervical region the cord segments and vertebral level matches while in upper dorsal region the cord segment is two less than the vertebral level i.e. D_2 segment of the cord will be opposite D_4 vertebra. In lower dorsal the difference is of three, meaning the D_8 segment of the cord will be in relation to D_{11} vertebra. In lumbar area there are fixed bony landmarks. L_3 cord segment is opposite D_{11} vertebra, S_1 cord segment is opposite D_{12} vertebra. The conus the lowest end of the cord is opposite the lower border of L_1 vertebra. The above-mentioned relationship is very important for precise localization in paraplegic patients.

Spinal nerves are 'mixed nerves' and. they contain both afferent and efferent fibres. Afferent fibres enter the cord via dorsal root, which breaks into numerous rootlets before entering the cord. Ventral root contains efferent fibres, which are axons of anterior horn cells. Dorsal root ganglia located on the dorsal root contain 1st order neurones of afferent fibres. Radical or root is a proximal portion of spinal nerve and the term radiculopathy is used to refer to a disease of spinal root.

'Cauda-Equina' is term used to describe the bunch of lumbar and sacral roots descending down from lower part of spinal cord exiting at their respective intervertebral foramina. 'Conus medullaris' is the lower most part of the cord. It consists of S_3-S_5 segments Filum terminale is a thin, slender, non-nervous filament and attaches to the dural sac at the level of second sacral vertebra.

CROSS-SECTIONAL ANATOMY OF CORD

Transverse section of Spinal cord

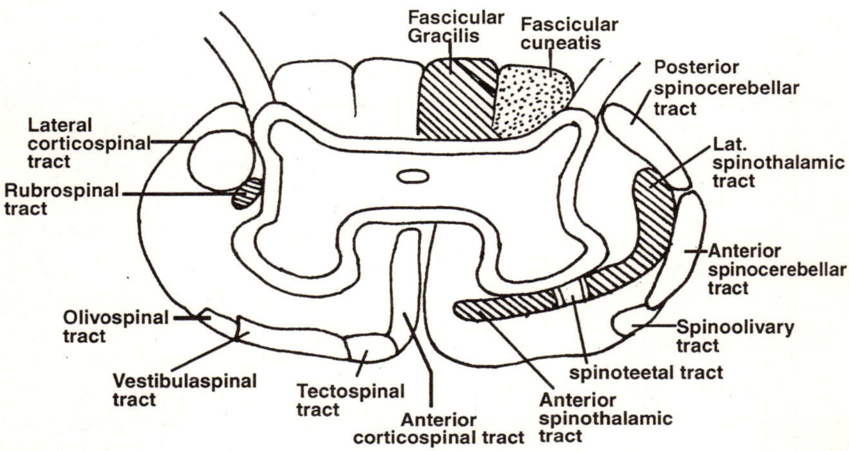

Fig 3.4: Cross-section of spinal cord and various tracts

Above diagram shows the centrally placed grey matter, shaped like an 'H', which divides the white matter into dorsal, lateral and anterior funiculus. A laminar architecture of nine cell layers or laminae can be distinguished within the grey matter. Zone of Lissauer separates the dorsal grey column from the surface of the spinal cord.

Table 3.5

Some Special Nuclear Columns Of Spinal Cord

Column	Location
Substantia gelatinosa (Laminae II)	C_1-S_5
Nucleus dorsalis	C_8-L_2 or L_3
Intermedio-lateral cell column	T_1-L_2 or L_3
Sacral autonomic nucleus	S_2-S_4

WHITE MATTER OF SPINAL CORD

The whiter matter of the spinal cord consists of myelinated and unmyelinated nerve fibres, which, are arranged, in longitudinal bundles or fasciculus. Tracts are defined as bundle of nerve fibres with the same origin and function. Dorsal column contains Fasciculus gracilis (medially) and Fasciculus cuneatus (laterally). They are concerned with proprioceptive and other fine discriminatory sensory information from the ipsilateral side of the body.

Lateral fasciculus has both ascending and descending tracts Lateral cortico-spinal tract is the most important descending tract, which is concerned with fine motor control. Medial reticulo-spinal tract originates from medullary reticular formation and is inhibitory to the stretch reflexes and flexor withdrawal reflexes of the spinal cord. Incomplete cord transaction such as demyelination involves medial reticulo-spinal tract in the lateral fasciculus. This leads to profound spasticity and paraplegia in extension due to unopposed action of vestibulo-spinal tract located in anterior funiculus. The vestibulo-spinal tract is facilitatory for stretch reflexes.

Lateral spino-thalamic tracts carry pain and temperature sensations from contralateral side of the body. Lamination in the tract is such that fibres from lower parts of body are located laterally. This forms the basis of sacral sparing with slowly progressing intramedullary lesions and early involvement of sacral sensations with extramedullary compression. Most laterally in the lateral fasciculus are the spino-cerebellar tracts concerned with unconscious proprioceptive sensations from muscle spindles and joints carried to the ipsilateral cerebellum.

Anterior fasciculus is located between ventral grey horn and anterior median fissure. This contains anterior cortico-spinal tract, which is functionally related to lateral cortico-spinal tract. The anterior fasciculus also contains vestibulo-spinal and anterior reticulo-spinal tracts, which are important for facilitatory influence on spinal stretch reflexes. Complete cord transaction leads to paraplegia in flexion due to release of flexor withdrawal reflexes, which are normally controlled by vestibulo-spinal tracts.

VASCULAR SUPPLY OF SPINAL CORD

Following are the main arteries:

1. Anterior spinal artery is formed by the midline union of paired branches of the vertebral arteries and descends along the median surface of cord, as a single vessel. At each segment it gives rise to anterior sulcal artery, which pierces the cord and supplies anterior 2/3rd of the cord.

2. Posterior spinal arteries are two in number, which arise from vertebral artery and course on the postero-lateral aspect of the cord. They supply the remaining 1/3rd of the cord. Anastamotic vessels connect the two 'arterial cornua' and supply the lateral side of the cord.

3. Radicular arteries arise from the intercostal arteries from T_1 to L_1 vertebral levels. These segmental branches re-enforce the vascular supply of the cord. Largest among them is at D_{10} called artery of Adamkewicz. These segmental branches are less in number in thoracic region thus making it prone to vascular insults. Moreover thoracic area comes in the watershed territory.

An irregular external venous plexus lying in epidural space surrounds the cord, draining ultimately into the vena cava.

PARAPLEGIA: It means paralysis of both lower limbs while the word paraparesis stands for less than complete weakness. Paraplegia can result from lesions involving upper spinal cord or lower motor neurons. For general usage, the term paraplegia is used for spinal cord pathologies, namely myelopathies. According to the speed of development of maximum deficit, paraplegia can be classified into

'Acute'	Maximum deficit within 48 hours
Subacute	Maximum deficit within 6 weeks
Chronic	Progressive weakness beyond 6 weeks

Table 3.6

Causes Of Paraplegia

Acute Paraplegia:

1. Infective	Acute transverse myelitis, Pott's spine Epidural abscess
2. Traumatic	
3. Vascular	Anterior spinal artery thrombosis, Hematomyelia, Epidural Haemorrhage
4. Neoplastic	Epidural metastasis

Subacute: (< 6 Wks)

1. Extramedullary compression of cord:

Aetiologies:
Infective: Pott's spine, Epidural abscess
Neoplastic : Metastasis, Lymphoma, Sarcoma

2. Intramedullary noncompressive lesions
   Aetiologies :
   Demyelination or multiple sclerosis
   Subacute combined degeneration

Chronic (> 6 Wks)

1. Degenerative aetiologies (non compressive)
   Hereditary spastic paraplegia – 4 autosomal dominant types, 2 recessive types and 2 X-linked recessive types.
   Motor neurone disease
   Adrenomyeloneuropathy
   Primary lateral sclerosis

2. Toxin mediated
   Lathyrism/Konzo

3. Compressive: Extramedullary : Pott's spine / Arachnoiditis, Spondylosis, Prolapse disc Neurofibroma / Meningioma, Atlanto-axial dislocation
   Intramedullary : Syringomyelia, Tumours

Various aetiologies, leading to paraplegia can also be divided according to the syndrome they cause.

1. Complete spinal cord section - Transverse myelopathy
2. Hemisection of spinal cord - Brown - Sequard syndrome.
3. Central cord syndrome
4. 'Pure motor' progressive myelopathy
5. Syndrome of dorsal column dysfunction with cortico spinal dysfunction
6. Anterior spinal artery syndrome

1. COMPLETE SPINAL CORD TRANSECTION

Commonest example is acute viral transverse myelitis where in all modalities of sensation are lost below the level of lesion, lower motor neurone signs are seen at the level of lesion, upper motor neurone type of weakness occurs below the level of the lesion.

Initially patient can be in 'Spinal shock' and. all activities below the level of lesion are suspended due to lack of supraspinal inputs. Sphincter involvement is common. Long-standing lesions cause either paraplegia in flexion or paraplegia in extension. Demyelinating lesions of the cord such as Multiple Sclerosis can also lead to spinal cord transaction but is usually incomplete and asymmetric unlike viral transverse myelitis, which is complete and symmetrical.

2. BROWN SEQUARD SYNDROME :

Brown-Sequard syndrome occurs due to lesion in one half of the cord. There is ipsilateral loss of proprioceptive sensations, ipsilateral pyramidal weakness, contralateral impairment of pain, temperature 2-3 segments below the level of lesion and lower motor neurone features at the level of the lesion. The fine touch is intact, because both dorsal columns and spino-thalamic tracts carry it. In a right-sided lesion of the cord, the sensation will be affected on the left side of the body and the motor paralysis will occur on the right side. This is due to the fact that the pyramidal fibres decussate higher up approximately two to three segments above while the spino-thalamic fibres decussate in the cord immediately There is loss of pain and temperature on the side opposite to the lesion while weakness and spasticity occurs on the same side of the lesion. Above-mentioned syndrome is typical for extramedullary lesions like cord compression but is also seen with intramedullary lesions like demyelination.

3. CENTRAL CORD SYNDROME:

Lesions in the centre of the cord such as syringomyelia, or tumours produce characteristic constellation of signs. There is involvement of decussating spino-thalamic tracts leading to bilateral impairment of pain and temperature over the affected dermatomes called suspended sensory loss. There is also dissociated sensory loss, meaning one modality of sensation – pain, and temperature is lost, while the fine touch is intact as both dorsal columns and anterior spino-thalamic tracts carry it. Dorsal column sensations (i.e. proprioception) remain intact. Sensations in the sacral region are spared. Affection of anterior horn cells leads to flaccid paralysis of upper limbs. Spastic paralysis of lower limbs is seen due to involvement of the pyramidal tracts.

4. PURE MOTOR PROGRESSIVE MYELOPATHY

It is due to predominant degeneration of cortico-spinal tracts as seen in Hereditary spastic paraplegia, Lathyrism, Adrenomyeloneuropathy, HTLV 1 associated myelopathy, Primary lateral sclerosis and Central disc herniation.

5. SYNDROME OF AFFECTION OF DORSAL COLUMNS AND CORTICOSPINAL TRACTS

The classic example is subacute combined degeneration, which is due to vitamin B_{12} deficiency. Patient presents with difficulty in gait, which becomes exaggerated when visual clues are lost, either when the eyes are closed, or in darkness. This is due to impaired proprioceptive sensations. Spasticity in the lower limbs is associated. It is important to diagnose this condition early, as it is treatable. Another example is HIV - induced vacuolar myelopathy. Arnold-Chairi malformation can also present in similar manner.

6. SYNDROME OF ANTERIOR SPINAL ARTERY THROMBOSIS

The clinical features are, acute lower limb weakness with a sensory level, sphincter involvement and intact proprioception as posterior spinal arteries supply posterior 1/3rd of cord.

When dealing with an upper motor neuron lesion resulting from a spinal cord disease, following points help to differentiate between the intrinsic and the extrinsic cord compressions. This distinction is important.

INTRAMEDULLARY AND EXTRAMEDULLARY LESIONS

Spinal cord tumours can be either intramedullary or extramedullary. Both can produce slowly progressive spasticity and weakness. Certain clinical guidelines, as mentioned in the Table3.7 can help to distinguish the two. Most notable is the dissociated sensory loss (fine touch dissociated from pain and temperature) seen with intramedullary lesions. Soft touch, carried by both dorsal column and anterior spino-thalamic tracts remains intact while pain and temperature senses are lost. Sacral sparing is also seen with intramedullary lesions as the sacral fibres are located most laterally in the spinothalamic tract and so do not get involved early in intramedullary lesions for example in intramedullary tumours like astrocytoma, ependymoma and syringomyelia. Extramedullary tumours can be either intradural or extradural. Intradural tumours arise from meninges, nerve roots, connective tissues and blood vessels such as meningioma, neurofibroma, lipoma, dermoids, hemangiomas, and metastasis. Extradural lesions like Pott's spine, tumours like lymphoma, sarcoma, and myeloma lead to prominent vertebral pain, which typically is more during recumbent decubitus (i.e. at night). Both intra and extradural lesions can lead to Brown - Sequard Syndrome.

Table3.7

Differentiation Of Intra And Extramedullary Lesions

	Intramedullary lesions	Extramedullary lesions
Type of pain	Funicular pain (Dull, aching pain, ill defined, distant from the site of the lesion).	Radicular and vertebral pain. Often severe at night, during recumbency.
Sensory loss	Dissociate sensory loss	Contralateral loss of pain and temperature with ipsilateral loss of proprioception
Sensory level	Rare	Coomon
Motor deficit	Wasting and diffuse extensive weakness	Localized weakness and wasting
Sacral sensations	Spared	Lost early
Trophic changes	Common	Uncommon
Progression	Descending	Ascending

COMPRESSIVE LESIONS OF THE SPINAL CORD

Compression of the cord can occur due to malformations of the vertebral canal like stenosis, and lesions of the vertebrae – both cancerous and non-cancerous. It can also occur due to a prolapsed intervertebral disc, tumours and granulomas of the meninges, tumours arising from the nerve roots and tumours and cysts, including syringomyelia, arising within the cord.

The compression can occur by lesions situated either, extradurally, intradullary or intramedullary.

Table 3.8

Compressive Lesions

Extradural:	Atlanto-axial dislocation and other cranio-vertebral malformations Fractures of vertebrae, spondylolisthesis, and stenosis of the canal Prolapsed intervertebral disc. Granulomas in the vertebra. Metastasis from primary tumours (forms the largest number of extradural tumours). Multiple myeloma. Hodgkin's lymphoma Haemangiomas and other vascular tumours Schwannoma (though it occurs intradurally, frequently, both intra and extradural growth in the form of 'dumb-bell' may occur) Meningioma (it is also common intradurally, rarely an extradural variety has been seen). Extradural sarcoma Lipoma.
Intradural – Extra-medullary	Here the lesion lies within the dura but outside the cord Arachnoidal cysts Granulomas Scwannoma Meningioma — these are the commonest tumours in this location Metastasis from primary outside and from CNS Lipoma
Intradural - Intra-medullary	Granuloma Syringomyelia and Hydromyelia Neurenteric cysts Glioma Haemangioblastoma A-V malformation Schwanomma (rare tumour at this site) Metastasis Spinal dysraphism and lipoma.

SYMPTOMS AND SIGNS: The symptoms of cord compression differ depending on the site of compression such as extradural, extra or intramedullary and also according to its segmental level in the cord. Symptoms will vary according to the acuteness of lesion.

Spinal compression affects the cord in two respects:

1) Direct compression that interferes with conduction in the tracts in the cord and conduction within the roots.

2) Compression of the spinal arteries, the radicular arteries, and veins leading to ischaemia of the cord, in turn leads to oedema of the cord and consequent degeneration of the ganglion cells with demyelination of the nerve roots and spinal tracts. Hence, it is imperative to detect the compression early, so that immediate decompression will result in total recovery.

SYMPTOMS:

Pain is the first symptom. In both extradural and extramedullary compression, the pain occurs in the distribution of the involved nerve roots at the level of compression. In the dorsal region, the pain is designated as "girdle pain" as these roots supply the trunk. Coughing, sneezing and movements of the spinal column intensify the pain. Local pain in the spinal column may also be present and is most marked in the case of cauda equina compression. Burning dysesthesae and paraesthesias occur late in the course of the illness and tend to involve the perianal region and distal parts of the lower limbs due to compression of the spino-thalamic tract. Paraesthesias occur early with extramedullary compression.

Motor symptoms appear soon after, from progression of the compressive lesion, due to pressure on the pyramidal tracts. The patients complain of stiffness of the lower limbs followed by weakness of the muscles of the pelvic girdle. Weakness is first noticed in climbing stairs, or while getting up from a low position such as squatting. Walking long distances or running becomes difficult. Motor symptoms occur early in extradural and intramedullary lesions. The weakness progresses to a spastic paralysis with patients complaining of flexor spasms.

Sphincter disturbances develop very late in extramedullary lesions with hesitancy and retention of urine. Constipation develops in some patients and persists through out the course of the disease. Intramedullary lesions tend to involve the sphincters early as compared to extramedullary lesions.

Signs: Signs of cord compression are discussed under the headings of motor signs, sensory signs, local and autonomic changes. Motor signs: Early involvement of the anterior roots especially in the cervical and lumbar regions leads to weakness and wasting of the muscles supplied by the affected roots. The C_5 root supplies the deltoids, C_6 the biceps and flexors of the wrist, C_{7-8} supply the triceps and extensors of the wrist while C_8 and T_1 supply the small muscles of the hand. The flexors of the hips are supplied by L_3 root, L_4 root supplies the peronei while L_5 and S_1 roots supply the elevators of the foot. L_5 and S_{1-3} roots supply the gastrocnemius, hamstrings and glutei. Fasciculation are also known to occur in root involvement.

Compression of the corticospinal tract leads to spasticity and weakness of the lower limbs. As the disease progresses and the compression intensifies, total paraplegia may develop. Initially there is paraplegia in extension followed by paraplegia in flexion. In high cervico-medullary junction compression (cranio-vertebral anomalies) weakness first appears in either upper extremity, followed by a clockwise or anticlockwise progression of weakness in the other three extremities. For example if the weakness first appears in the right arm, it is followed by weakness in right leg, then left leg and finally left arm leading to quadriparesis (Eisberg's phenomenon).

Sensory signs: Compression of the posterior root produces hyperaesthesia and hyperalgesia in the distribution of the involved nerve root. Roughly, C_5 root supplies the sensation in the skin over deltoid and tip of the thumb. Sensation by C_6 root is distributed in the antero-lateral region over the biceps and tip of index finger. C_7 root supplies the skin over antero-lateral aspect of the forearm and the tip of middle finger while the C_8 root supplies the medial aspect of the forearm and tips of ring and little fingers. T_1 and T_2 roots supply the sensation over the remaining medial area of forearm and arm.

In the lower limb the anterior aspect of thigh up to knee is supplied by L_3 root. The L_4 root supplies the medial aspect of the leg and extends over to lateral aspect of the foot. The lateral aspect of the leg and part of the foot is supplied by L_5 root. S_{1-3} roots supply the posterior aspect of the ankle, the leg and thigh inclusive of buttocks. And S_{4-5} roots supply the perianal region.

Compression of the spino-thalamic tracts leads to loss of pain and temperature sensations below and opposite to the side of the lesion. Touch is spared as it has double pathway in the cord. This leads to dissociated anaesthesia. Impairment of the joint position and vibration sense occurs early if the compression of the cord is situated posteriorly. (Fig. 4.2 and 4.3)

Locally, there is tenderness of the spine in extra and intra dural compression but is rare in the intramedullary lesions. When the patient flexes the neck a wave of paraesthesia may descend in the body (Lhermitte's sign). It may be seen in any lesion that involves the posterior column such as cervical spondylotic myelopathy. Spasms of the spinal muscles at the level of the lesion may result in limitation of movements of the spine. Finally, spinal scoliosis may be noted if the muscle spasm is unilateral.

Reflexes: The reflex are subserved by the root or segment of the cord involved is broken. Hence, the tendon reflex dependent on the affected root or segment is lost while the reflexes below the level of lesion are exaggerated. The plantar reflexes are extensor and the cremastric and abdominal reflexes are diminished or abolished. In a C_6 root or segmental lesion the biceps jerk will be abolished while the triceps jerk and lower limb reflexes are exaggerated. Inversion of the reflex occurs due to overflow phenomenon in the affected spinal segment. In case of biceps jerk, the overflow involves the flexors of the fingers and/or triceps, so that, on trying to elicit the biceps tendon reflex, there is no contraction of the biceps muscle but the fingers still flex or the arm may extend because of the contraction of triceps.

The autonomic changes are of poor localising value. However, excessive sweating may occur below the level of compression.

It is important to localise cord compression at cervical, thoracic, lumbar or sacral levels. The principles that govern such a localisation are detailed below.

At the level of lesion the anterior horn cells or the root will be compressed and damaged giving signs and symptoms of lower motor neurone involvement in the form of wasting, weakness and at times fasciculations. For example, involvement at the first dorsal level, will give rise to weakness and wasting of small muscles of the hand, whilst a lesion of the fifth lumbar segment will cause a foot drop. Thoracic level lesions may go unnoticed by the patient and can only be spotted by a diligent examiner. Intercostal wasting may be observed. Appropriate tendon reflexes are absent so that a lesion at fifth cervical segment will cause absence of biceps jerk.

Upper motor neurone involvement produces a spastic paraplegia leading to symptoms of stiffness of both lower limbs and inability to walk on uneven ground and difficulty in climbing stairs. With increasing spasticity the gait becomes markedly stiff. Examination at an early stage may reveal only a minimal increase in tone with brisk reflexes. The abdominal reflexes will be absent while the plantar response will be extensor. As the compression increases the spasticity becomes more pronounced and patellar and ankle clonus may be elicited. Weakness due to a pyramidal lesion usually appears first in the extensor group of muscles in the upper extremity and flexor group of muscles in the lower extremities. Therefore shoulder abduction, elbow extension, wrist extension and finger abduction will be weak in the upper extremity while in the lower extremity, hip flexion, knee flexion and dorsiflexion of the foot will be weaker.

Pain results from nerve root compression and may be dull aching, shooting or knife-like. At times hyperaesthesia occurs and the patient may describe the area as "sore" or as if "a sand paper has been rubbed on it". The pain generally extends from the back along a given dermatome (girdle pain in dorsal region).

Damage to the spino-thalamic tracts and posterior columns produces symptoms of tingling and numbness. Deep dull aching pains or shearing pain or cold feeling result from spino-thalamic involvement. Patients may state that they get a feeling as if they are walking on soft ground – cotton wool. The pain and temperature sensation is diminished or absent below the level of lesion. Touch sensation is usually preserved as it has dual pathway. The joint position sense at toes may be impaired if the dorsal columns are affected. Similarly vibration sense may also be impaired below the level of the lesion.

Below is the brief review of features of individual segmental involvement at different levels.

Cervical $_1$ to $_4$: Patients will complain of upper nuchal pain with stiffness in neck movements. The pain may extend to supra-clavicular region in C_4 lesion. A spastic quadriparesis with a clockwise spread of weakness and a sensory level extending up to clavicle and involving both upper extremities is seen. This clinical picture is seen with cranio-vertebral junction anomalies especially with chronic atlanto-axial dislocation. Joint position sense may be lost in all four extremities. Occasionally, wasting and weakness of small muscles of the hands is seen with atlanto-axial dislocation and is thought to be due to involvement of the anterior spinal artery. In platybasia, (basilar invagination) due to presence of a small size posterior fossa, signs of involvement of the lower cranial nerves either unilateral or bilateral and signs of cerebellar involvement are present. Arnold-Chairi malformation (herniation of tonsils in foramen magnum) and syringomyelia may accompany the platybasia. In cranio-vertebral anomalies the neck is short and the hair-line is low. (Fig. 3. 5).

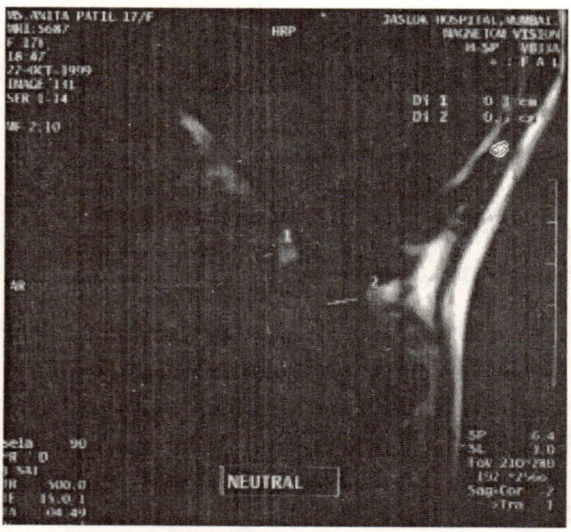

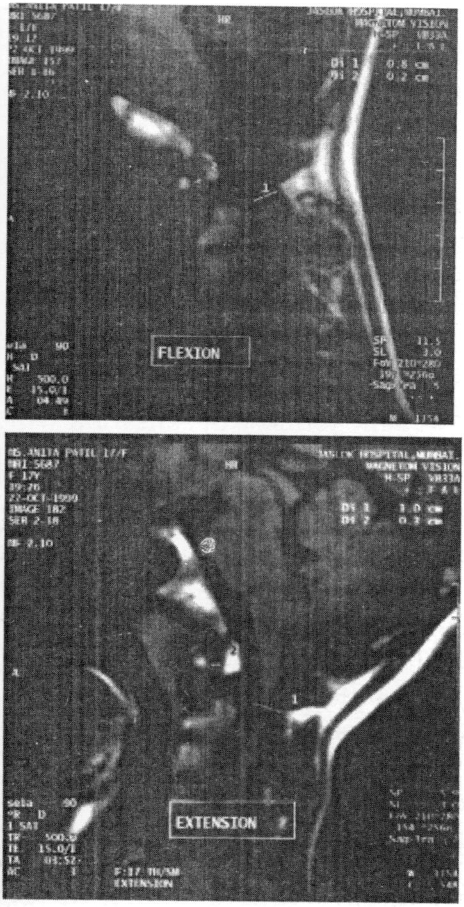

Fig. 3.5. MRI - Cranio vertebral anomaly. Seperation of odontoid from C2. Partial fusion of C2-C3. Posterior angulation of C2 with considerable indentation on cervical subarachnoid space & cord. Thinning of cervical cord at C1-C2 level with altered signal intensity. Focal hypointense areas within the cord on T1 weighted images - Myelomalacia. No significant change in flexion & extension.

Cervical $_5$ and $_6$: Pain and loss of sensation occurs along the lateral border of the arm in (C_5) and forearm to thumb in (C_6) lesion. The deltoid, supraspinatus, infraspinatus, rhomboids, biceps and brachioradialis muscles are weak. The biceps and supinator reflexes are absent or inverted. The triceps, knee and ankle jerks are exaggerated. The abdominal and cremasteric reflexes are absent and the plantar response is extensor. The sensory level is anywhere below the clavicle depending on the damage caused to the pathways by the compressing lesion. In a fully evolved lesion the sensory level is at the level of clavicle.

Cervical $_{7,8}$ and Dorsal$_1$: Pain and loss of sensation will extend from the axilla (D_1) to the triceps (C_7) and medial forearm region including the little and ring fingers (C_8). The triceps jerk will be absent and biceps and supinator jerks will be normal. The other signs and symptoms are similar to a lesion at C_5 region.

Dorsal $_2$ to Dorsal$_7$: Pain and hyperaesthesia or loss of sensation occurs in the region of the dermatome involved (girdle pains). The sensory level will be three segments below the level of compression. That is, if the fourth dorsal segment is involved, the sensory level will be anywhere below the D_7 level. Spastic paraplegia will be present.

Dorsal $_8$ to $_{10}$ and Dorsal $_{10}$ to $_{12}$: Pain and loss of sensation will depend on the dermatome involved. Weakness can be demonstrated in the upper abdominal muscles in D $_8$ to $_{10}$ lesions. If the examiner asks the patient to lift the head and trunk off the bed, while lying supine, the umbilicus will be dragged downwards, due to non-contraction of the upper abdominal muscles and normal contraction of the lower abdominal muscles. In D $_{10}$ to $_{12}$ lesions the reverse occurs and the umbilicus moves upwards. The sensory level and pyramidal involvement follow the pattern of upper thoracic level compressions except the sensory level is two segments below the segment involved.

LESIONS OF CAUDA-EQUINA AND CONUS MEDULLARIS

Cauda Equina consists of bundles of lumbar, sacral and coccygeal nerve roots that pass caudally from their cord attachments to exit at their appropriate intervertebral foramina. Conus medullaris is the cone shaped termination of the spinal cord at lower border of L_1 vertebra. It consists of spinal cord segments S_3-S_5. Lesions of cauda-equina lead to asymmetric, areflexic, flaccid paralysis with radicular pains, impaired perineal, thigh and leg sensation and sphincter disturbances. At the level of D_{12}-L_1 vertebrae, compression of the 'epiconus' (i.e. cord just above the conus) can lead to an extensor Babinski sign and a spastic bladder, in addition to the other features mentioned above. Conus lesions usually lead to symmetric, saddle anaesthesia with early sphincter disturbances. In reality there is neither any practical utility in separating cauda and conus lesions nor do they exist in pure forms.

Table 3.9

Differentiation Of Conus Medullaris And Cauda Equina Lesions

	Conus medullaris	**Cauda Equina**
Motor weakness	Symmetric, mild No fasciculation	Asymmetric, severe Fasciculation in paralysed muscles
Sensory loss	Saddle anaesthesia symmetric Dissociated sensory loss	Over thigh, leg, buttock No dissociation
Radicular pains	Uncommon	Very common
Sphincter disturbances	Early & marked	Late and less marked
Deep tendon reflexes	Ankle jerks may be lost knee jerks present	Knee and ankle jerks both are absent
Sexual functions	Early and prominent	Late and mild
Trophic changes	Common	Less common
Causes (common)	Tumours (Ependymoma) Tethered cord	Prolapsed disc Tumours (neurofibroma) Infections, Metastasis Trauma Diabetic radiculopathy

The common lesions of the conus medullaris are ependymoma and spinal dysraphism (a dermoid or lipoma). The lower sacral roots are involved leading to pain in the perianal and genital regions. The sensations in these areas are diminished. The male patient may complain of impotency and the female may complain of loss of libido. Low back pain is common and dribbling incontinence almost always occurs. The anal reflex is absent. The knee jerks are brisk but the ankle jerks may be lost, with a foot drop. If the extensors of toes are spared, the Babinski response may be elicited.

Cauda equina lesion may be either medial or lateral.

Lateral cauda equina lesion: The usual lesion of a lateral cauda equina is a neurofibroma or a lumbar disc prolapse. Pain in the anterior thigh, with diminution or loss of sensation in the distribution of L_2 and L_3 dermatome is noted. The quadriceps muscle is weak and the knee jerk is absent due to L_{2-3} roots being involved. If there is pressure on the conus, the ankle jerk may be brisk with an extensor plantar response. A large disc extrusion may even cause sphincter incontinence.

Middle or medial cauda equina lesion: This leads to bilateral lumbar and sacral roots involvement with pain along both sciatic nerves. Weakness and wasting of the muscles of the feet along with involvement of the hamstrings and glutei is noted. The knee jerk may be preserved or brisk due to weakness of the hamstrings. The ankle jerk is absent. Sensory loss involves appropriate dermatomes. Apart from disc prolapse, lipomas and tethering of the cord, the tumours that produce this type of lesions are chordomas, metastatic tumours, leukaemic infiltrates or seeding from a medulloblastoma of the posterior fossa.

To establish the cause of compression, one needs to do the following investigations. Routine blood counts, ESR, serum biochemistry and rarely specialised investigations for leukaemia, myeloma etc.

Before the advent of CAT scan, routine roentgenogram of the spine was always a very helpful investigation. It still can throw light on infective process, deposits etc. CSF examination although not diagnostic is still indicated. Infective process, leukaemic deposits etc. will be reflected in the routine CSF examination. Rise in protein, xanthochromia and positive Queckenstedt's test will suggest spinal compression. Failure of rise in CSF pressure on jugular compression indicates subarachnoid block. Scanning, either a CAT scan or MRI scan is today the most important investigation to establish the cause of compression and also the level of compression. SPECT scan will help to establish whether other bones of the body are also involved. Surgery is the treatment for all compressive lesions. The type and extent of surgery will depend on the pathology of the lesion.

Table 3.10

Correlation Of Spinal Segments Involved With Clinical Features

Level of lesion	Symptoms & signs	Muscles affected	Reflexes
Above C_5	Nuchal pain Quadriplegia	Trapezius, Pectorals Diaphragm	All brisk
C_5-C_6	Pain and loss of sensation in the lateral border of arm & forearm, paraplegia and sensory level below clavicle	Deltoids, biceps brachio-radialis supra & infra spinati	Biceps & supinator lost or inverted other reflexes very brisk
C_7- T_1	Pain and loss of sensation from axilla to triceps, medial forearm and ring & little finger, paraplegia, sensory level below clavicle	Triceps, small muscles of hand	Biceps & supinator normal & triceps lost knee & ankle brisk
D_{2-7}	Girdle pains sensory level 3 segments below level of lesion, paraplegia	Intercostals	Knee & ankle brisk
D_{8-10}	Same as above	Upper abdominals weak	Loss of upper abdominal reflexes KJ & AJ brisk
D_{10-12}	Same as above	Lower abdominals weak	Loss of lower abdominal reflexes, KJ & AJ brisk
L_{2-3}	Inguinal pain, minimal spasticity	Weakness quadriceps	Knee jerk lost
Conus medullaris	Saddle anaesthesia, incontinence	Sphincters weak	AJ absent
Cauda equina	Radicular pain incontinence rare	Asymmetric foot muscle weakness hamstrings, glutei	KJ & AJ absent

Table 3.11

Differentiation Between Extradural, Intradural And Intra-Medullary Lesions

	Extradural	Intradural	Intramedullary
Pain- root Distribution	+	+	-
Pain, Local	+	+/-	-
Paraesthesae	Early	Early-	
Sensory loss	Rising level	Rising level	Dissociated loss
Weakness	First -	Later than sensory	Early
Fasciculation & atrophy	+/-	+/-	++
Sphincter	Late	Late	Early
Trophic changes	+/-	+/-	+

At times, the spinal cord diseases may be associated with radicular or peripheral nerve involvement and then the following differential diagnoses need to be considered.

Table 3.12

Myeloradiculopathies And Myeloneuropathies

Myeloradiculopathy	Myeloneuropathy
Tubercular arachnoiditis	Subacute combined degeneration
Neurosyphilis	Adrenomyeloneuropathy
Fungal meningitis	Metachromatic leukodystrophy
Lyme disease	Krabbe's disease
Malignant infiltrations	Central peripheral distal axonopathy
Cervical spondylotic process	e.g. hexacarbon toxicity
	Subacute myelo-optic neuropathy
	Systemic lupus erythematosus
	Hereditary spastic paraplegia

MICTURITION AND BLADDER DYSFUNCTION

The function of the lower urinary tract is storage and voluntary expulsion of urine. The urinary bladder has smooth muscle divided into trigone and the detrusor. The internal sphincter, which has smooth muscle, and the external sphincter having the striated muscle maintain normal continence. The striated external urethral sphincter is supplied by the somatic fibres from the pudendal nerves (S_{2-4}). The sympathetic nerve inflow to the bladder comes from T_{11} to L_2 segments. The body has beta-receptors and the sphincter has alpha-receptors, so the stimulation of the sympathetic nerves results in relaxation of the body of the bladder and simultaneous contraction of the bladder neck, resulting in bladder filling. The parasympathetic supply comes from S_{2-4} segments and parasympathetic stimulation leads to sustained contraction of the detrusor leading to emptying of bladder. Thus, sympathetic nerves are for filling and the parasympathetic nerves are for emptying. Normal micturition is a result of coordination between the sympathetic and the parasympathetic nerves.

Following centres and reflex arcs control the storage and smooth evacuation of urine.

1. **SPINAL REFLEX ARCS:**

A) **DETRUSOR REFLEX ARC:** Afferents are the visceral afferent fibres which carry the sensation from stretch receptors in bladder wall to the sacral cord segments S_2-S_4 ('Detrusor nuclei'). The efferents are the preganglionic parasympathetic fibres from S_{2-4} enter pelvic nerves and relay in the ganglia located in the detrusor muscle itself. Postganglionic nerves then innervate the muscles. This is the main arc for affecting the parasympathetic mediated detrusor contraction.

B) **URETHRAL REFLEX ARC:** The afferents are the visceral afferents from external urethra and travel through the pudendal motor neurons S_{2-4} (also called Onuf's nucleus). Efferents are from the pudendal nerve, a somatic nerve, which stimulates the striated sphincter i.e. external urethral sphincter contraction via nicotinic receptors. This reflex maintains the urethral pressure higher than intravesical pressure during storage phase, thus facilitating storage.

2. **BRAINSTEM MICTURITION CENTRE:** is situated in the pontine tegmentum. It controls the detrusor and urethral reflex arcs and maintains the detrusor-sphincter synergy during voiding.

3. **CEREBRAL CORTEX:** Right inferior frontal gyrus and right anterior cingulate gyrus are involved in the micturition process. These centres judge the social appropriateness of the act of micturition and order the pontine centre accordingly. These centres can also stop the ongoing micturition by its direct control over pudendal motor neurons S_{2-4}.

4. **ROLE OF SYMPATHETIC:** Sympathetic outflow for bladder arises from D_{10}-L_2 and its stimulation leads to inhibition of detrusor contraction via beta-receptors and contraction of internal urethral sphincter via alpha-receptors thus helping the storage of urine. Sensory afferents from bladder enter the sacral cord. Till 400-600 ml of urine accumulates, the intravesical pressure is less than urethral pressure, maintained by urethral reflex arc, and so the detrusor does not contract. But beyond that, intravesical pressure rises and the detrusor starts to contract through the detrusor reflex arc. This is soon inhibited by the pontine centre, which receives bladder afferents, ascending to it in the lateral funiculus of cord. The centre, in addition, also re-enforces the urethral reflex arc.

During voiding phase, cerebral cortex initially assesses the social appropriateness and then stimulates the pontine centre, which then releases the detrusor reflex and maintains the detrusor sphincter synergy to facilitate smooth urination.

NEUROGENIC BLADDER

Neurogenic bladder is defined as bladder dysfunction due to neurological lesions. It can be classified broadly into the upper motor neuron type, which includes the uninhibited bladder and the automatic bladder. The lower motor neuron type includes sensory neurogenic, motor neurogenic and autonomous neurogenic bladder.

UNINHIBITED BLADDER: Lesions rostral to pontine centre especially frontal lobe tumours, and normal pressure hydrocephalus result in uninhibited bladder.

Characteristics:

1. Sensation of bladder fullness: Normal

2. Urgency, frequency, urge incontinence and patient would feel surprised and embarrassed by the incontinence
3. Voiding is started normally
4. No hesitancy due to normal detrusor sphincter synergy
5. No residual urine

AUTOMATIC OR SPASTIC BLADDER: Lesion between pontine centre and sacral cord such as multiple sclerosis and cord compression result in automatic bladder.

Characteristics :

1. Sensations may be decreased or normal.
2. Urgency, frequency, urge incontinence.
3. Difficulty in initiating to void.
4. Hesitancy, retention due to detrusor sphincter dysynergia.
5. Mild to moderate residual urine.

LOWER MOTOR NEURONE BLADDER: Three types can be identified.

I. **AUTONOMOUS:** Lesions at conus medullaris or detrusor areflexia due to tumours

Features:

1. Absent bladder sensation.
2. Distension of bladder due to lack of detrusor tone.
3. Over flow incontinence.
4. Inability to void.
5. Associated saddle anaesthesia.
6. High residual urine.

II. **SENSORY:** Lesion in afferent pathway, as in. tabes dorsalis, syringomyelia, or diabetes.

Features: Same as above except that voiding ability will be intact

III. **MOTOR:** Lesions in efferent pathway e.g. Myelomeningocoele, Diabetes, Lumbar canal stenosis.
Features: Same as above except that there will be painful retention of urine.

CHAPTER IV

CEREBELLAR AND SENSORY SYSTEM

CEREBELLAR ANATOMY :

Cerebellum comprises of midline vermis and two lateral cerebellar hemispheres formed by the Anterior lobe (paleocerebellum), Posterior lobe (neocerebellum) and Flocculonodular lobe (archicerebellum). Cerebellar lobes are divided by fissures into lobules, which are in turn divided into folia. Each folium is composed of cerebellar cortex with a strip of white matter. Cerebellar cortex is divided into 3 layers from outside to inside, the molecular layer, purkinje cell layer and the granular layer. Purkinje cells are the most important cells and are responsible for the output of cerebellar cortex. In the white matter lie the four pairs of deep nuclei, the fastigial nucleus (most medial), globose and emboli forming a nucleus also called nucleus interpositus and the most lateral dentate nucleus.

Three cerebellar peduncles attach the cerebellum to the brainstem. The inferior peduncle mainly contains afferent fibres to cerebellum like spino-cerebellar and vestibulo-cerebellar tracts, middle peduncle relays the ponto cerebellar afferent fibres from contralateral pontine nuclei and superior peduncle is the efferent peduncle and carries the efferent tracts from deep cerebellar nuclei to the thalamus and cortex.

PHYSIOLOGICAL CONSIDERATIONS:

Cerebellum controls the ipsilateral parts of the body. Functionally cerebellum can be divided into three components depending upon their afferent fibre connections. Flocculonodular lobe is also called vestibulo cerebellum as it receives special proprioceptive fibres from vestibular nuclei. Its function is maintenance of body equilibrium. Anterior lobe is also known as spinocerebellum as its main afferents are the spino-cerebellar tracts, which bring information from muscle spindles and joints. Its main function is to control posture and muscle tone. Posterior lobe receives ponto-cerebellar fibres and hence is called pontocerebellum. Its function is to co-ordinate skilled movements initiated at the cortical level.

But cerebellar function is hardly as simple as mentioned above. For better understanding, keeping in view both the efferent and afferent connections, it is better to divide the cerebellum in three longitudinal divisions rather than the transverse anatomical divisions mentioned above.

VERMIAN (MIDLINE) ZONE

Main function is the control of axial stability (equilibrium), eye movements and co-ordination of head and eye movements. Lesions of the vermian region lead to truncal ataxia, as seen in alcoholic cerebellar degeneration.

PARAVERMIAN (INTERMEDIATE) ZONE

Main function of this zone is to smoothly co-ordinate the 'ongoing' muscle activity. Dorsal and ventral spino-cerebellar tracts bring afferent information regarding the ongoing actual body movement to ipsilateral cerebellum. At the same time, the cerebellum is appraised of the central command issued for that movement through descending fronto-ponto-cerebellar tracts. Both commands are analysed in this zone and changes effected for smooth co-ordination of the movements, which are then fed back to the supplementary motor cortex by the efferent tracts via interpositus nuclei which exit through superior cerebellar peduncle.

Dorsal spino-cerebellar tracts provide precise information from the ipsilateral muscle spindles and Golgi tendon organs of leg and trunk muscles. Ventral spino-cerebellar tract after arising from spinal border cells, cross to opposite side and ascend to the level of superior cerebellar peduncle. They cross the midline again and enter the peduncle to relay in paravermian region. Lesions in paravermian region lead to ataxia of ipsilateral limbs, dysdiadokokinesis, that is inability to perform rapid alternating movements and intention tremor which is uncontrolled shaking of the fingers towards the end of the movement, on approaching the target.

LATERAL ZONE

It comprises of lateral hemispheres with the dentate nuclei. It receives information from supplementary and pre-motor cortex, and helps to initiate volitional movements. This is accomplished by dentato-rubro-thalamic tracts, which exit through superior cerebellar peduncles. Lesions of this region lead to delay in initiation of volitional activity.

CLINICAL FEATURES OF CEREBELLAR DISEASES:

Incoordination of Limbs: This is the most prominent manifestation of cerebellar disease, which is mainly due to lesions in the lateral hemispheres of the cerebellum. Following tests are done to elucidate the incoordination.

1. **Finger nose test:** With eyes open and arm held in full abduction, patient is told to touch his/her nose. Note for dysmetria (over or undershooting of limb) and intention tremor (side to side, rhythmic oscillations of finger as it approaches the target). Holmes tremor earlier called rubral tremor, is the term used for resting tremor of the hand, which is slow in frequency (< 4.5Hz) but markedly increases on action and has prominent intention component. It is seen with lesions of superior cerebellar peduncle.
2. **Heel-knee test:** Patient is asked to lift the heel of one leg and place it on opposite knee and then slide on the shin of that limb. Look for 'clumsiness' of performance and side-to-side movement of the limb.
3. **Dysdiadokokinesis:** means inability to perform rapid alternating movements. Patient is asked to hold his forearms vertically with palms facing inwards and rapidly rotate the hands and forearms at the elbow.
4. **Past pointing:** Patient sits opposite the examiner and is told to lift the arm up and touch the examiners outstretched index finger. With cerebellar disease, finger would deviate to ipsilateral side.

   A 3-4Hz rhythmic nodding of head (titubation): This is seen with vermian lesions.

Speech: Scanning dysarthria is a feature of cerebellar disease. Ask the patient to say 'Mumbai' and he will say M-U-M-B-A-I thus prolonging the time taken to say each syllable giving the scanning quality to the speech. When the speech changes in volume and the initial letters tend to be explosive, the speech is known as staccato speech.

Eye Signs : In cerebellar diseases, there is gaze-evoked nystagmus horizontally, with the fast component away from the midline. The nystagmus is more prominent and coarse on the side of the lesion. Nystagmus is elicited when the gaze is directed laterally. Dysmetria is seen with eyes in the central position. When the patient is asked to focus on an object in the midline, the eyes will make few oscillations before focus is achieved.

Gait disorder: With midline cerebellar lesions affecting the vermis, for example, medulloblastomas and alcoholic degeneration, patient develops truncal ataxia, i.e. walking like a drunkard. To unmask mild ataxia patient is asked to walk on a straight line (tandem walking), stand on one foot, walk backwards or hop in a small square.

Hypotonia: Tone is reduced in cerebellar disorders due to suppression of gamma and alpha motor neurone activity. This is seen more often with acute cerebellar lesions. To demonstrate hypotonia, hold the forearm vertically with elbow resting on table. If the wrist droops with the angle between forearm and wrist more than 70 degrees, hypotonia is inferred. Pendular knee jerk is another manifestation of hypotonia.With the patient sitting on the bed and legs hanging down, strike on the quadriceps tendon. Normally leg will extend and return two or three times. With cerebellar lesions, due to hypotonia, back and forth movements will continue for longer time like a pendulum of clock.

Holmes' rebound phenomenon: Ask the patient to flex his elbow against resistance and suddenly let go. Normally, the antagonist muscles would rapidly check the released flexion of the forearm. This does not happen in cerebellar diseases and the patient's hand might strike the chest with force.

DISEASES OF THE CEREBELLUM

CEREBELLAR MALDEVELOPMENT is usually due to DNA repair defects. It is often associated with the Dandy-Walker syndrome and the Arnold-Chiari malformation. In the Dandy-Walker syndrome the exit foramina of the ventricles, namely the foramen of Luschka and Magendie, which develop at the seventh week of gestation fail to open. It results in dilatation of the fourth ventricle, which enlarges, and leaves no space for the growing cerebellum. A massive midline cyst, the original fourth ventricle, develops instead, with atrophic cerebellar tissue lying besides the cyst. Signs of cerebellar lesions in infancy become apparent around two years of age, as the pyramidal pathways become functional, but there may be no symptom till as late as the second decade of life. The Dandy-Walker syndrome usually presents with signs of obstructive hydrocephalus, such as an enlarging head, headaches, vomiting and papilloedema.

The Arnold-Chiari malformation may be a result of pontine maldevelopment. The pontine flexure does not form and a part of cerebellum and medulla is pushed down in the cervical canal. The malformation becomes symptomatic at any time, from the age of two till late in the third decade of life. It may present with signs of an obstructive hydrocephalus, or with combinations of signs such as lower cranial nerve palsies, ataxia, spastic quadriparesis and deficits in proprioception involving the upper extremities. Abnormalities of the cranio-vertebral region, namely basilar invagination, occipitalisation of the atlas, maldevelopment of the atlas with atlanto-axial dislocation, etc. are often seen in our country. These conditions should always be remembered when one is examining a patient with cerebellar disease. A short neck and low hairline is observed with these conditions. Basilar invagination is associated with a small posterior fossa and herniation of tonsils into the upper cervical canal.

Ataxia resulting from progressive degeneration of the cerebellum and its connections can be idiopathic or hereditary. The idiopathic variety could be due to metabolic disorders, mitochondrial disorders or autoimmune.

METABOLIC DISORDERS: Many of the cerebellar diseases of childhood present as acute attacks that recur, and where no cause can be found. The child is free of symptoms after two or three attacks, which generally occur after first year of life and continue through out the first decade of life. An individual attack may last for a few days and recur within months or several years. Maple syrup urine disease, a disorder with increased amounts of Valine, Leucine and Isoleucine excreted in urine, is a fatal disease of childhood that may show cerebellar signs. Hartnup's disease, a disorder of tryptophan metabolism, has cerebellar signs, pellagra like skin, and peripheral neuropathy. Malabsorption of vitamin E may lead to ataxia.

Mitochondria in a cell have their own genome. A defect in the genome leads to defects of respiratory enzymes of the cell. Leigh's encephalopathy a mitochondrial genome defect leads to disorder of pyruvate metabolism, and is a cause of acute ataxia.

THE IMMUNE DISORDERS that lead to ataxia are Miller Fisher syndrome, a variant of Guillain Barre syndrome, multiple sclerosis and paraneoplastic cerebellar degeneration.

MULTIPLE SCLEROSIS is an important cause of cerebellar dysfunction. It can begin with visual loss due to demyelination in the optic nerve or optic tract. Signs of brainstem and spinal cord involvement may herald the onset of the disease. It usually presents in late twenties as a unilateral loss of vision in a female. The patient then has a relapsing and remitting course with spinal cord and cerebellar signs developing as the disease progresses. The initial loss of vision is rapid, with the vision reduced to mere perception of light or even total blindness, in matter of hours. This disease is called retrobulbar or optic neuritis and generally recovers completely. The ophthalmoscopic examination is initially normal, though later optic atrophy and Marcus-Gunn pupils develop. The patient complains of pain on moving the eyes. Spinal cord and brainstem dysfunction cause pyramidal signs, sphincter disturbances, diplopia and dysphagia. Uncommonly, there are some cases of multiple sclerosis that present with complete transaction of the cord, and others that show only brainstem involvement.

Over many years the unfortunate patient is left with substantial neurological deficit and is crippled by the disease. Death is generally due to intercurrent infections. The diagnosis is firmly established if there is a history of remission and relapses, and signs point to lesions in the neuraxis at various levels. CSF examination shows increase in gamma globulin with demonstration of oligoclonal bands and presence of myelin basic protein. Visual, auditory and somatosensory responses are abnormal in the vast majority. MRI shows evidence of demyelination at various sites. To confirm the diagnosis, at least five demyelinating plaques in the MRI should be demonstrated.

The aetiology of the disease is autoimmune in nature. It is a disease of temperate climate and affects people who live in the northern hemispheres. However, it is also seen in India.

Intravenous administration of 500 – 1000 mg. daily of Methylprednisolone during the acute attack for 5 to 7 days does cut short relapse and hastens recovery. Maintenance dose of Prednisolone and/or Azathioprin is also advocated when the attacks recur frequently. Interferon beta is being given to reduce the number of relapses. Recently, plasmapharesis once a month is being tried as interferon beta is very expensive and not available in India.

INFECTIVE DISORDERS: Ataxia sometimes follows acute viral infections such as chicken pox, measles, and infectious mononucleosis. It may follow within three to six weeks of infection and continue for a few months. Jakob-Cruetzfeldt disease, a prion disorder may present with ataxia.

THE HEREDITARY ATAXIAS form a very important group of ataxias in India. They are inherited as autosomal dominant, autosomal recessive or sex-linked. The common autosomal recessive ataxia, known as Friedreich's ataxia, is described below.

FRIEDREICH'S ATAXIA: It is an autosomal recessively inherited disorder. It is caused by expansions of 200-900 GAA trinucleotide repeats in the STM/X25 gene on the long arm of chromosome 9. The gene encodes the protein called frataxin, the function of which is still not well established. However, the greater the number of expansions, lesser the amount of frataxin formed, but there is phenotypic variability observed independently of the repeat length.

Nikolaus Friedreich described this form of ataxia around 1870. The onset of the disease is around 8-10 years of age or before 20 years of age. It usually begins as progressive gait disturbance with ataxia involving the upper limbs after a few years. Later speech is affected producing dysarthria within 5 years of onset of the disease. On examination the patient may have optic atrophy, deafness, nystagmus, staccato speech, ataxia and muscle weakness of all four limbs, brisk tendon reflexes in the upper limbs and absent knee and ankle jerks with extensor plantar responses. There is loss of position and vibration sense in the lower limbs. Kyphoscoliosis, pes cavus and hammer toes are present. There is cardiomyopathy of the hypertrophic non-obstructive type. The electrocardiogram shows prolongation of P-R interval, bundle branch block, and S-T segment changes. The EMG and nerve conduction studies show, axonal sensory neuropathy, with prolonged central motor and sensory conduction and prolonged or absent peripheral potentials of somato-sensory evoked potentials. In 1995, families with autosomal recessive ataxia linked to chromosome 9q13 have been found with later onset of the disease or retained knee and ankle reflexes.

THE DOMINANTLY INHERITED ATAXIA is of many genotype and phenotypes. They are commonly known as <u>spino-cerebellar ataxias (SCA).</u> Till date, 16 varieties have been described.

It is a heterogeneous group of neurodegenerative disorder affecting cerebellum and its connections. They are due to expansion of CAG repeat – in genetic terminology known as triplet repeat disease. Most of the recessive ataxias begin in the early childhood or teenage years. The initial symptom is progressive gait ataxia. Later the upper limbs and speech become involved. SCA 1,2,3, 6 and 7 usually start in early childhood. SCA 6 has also been described with late onset. SCA 6 is of early onset and rapid progress, due to defect in alpha A –voltage dependent calcium channel and have ataxia with action tremors and action myoclonus. SCA 4,5, and 10-14 usually have pure cerebellar degeneration. SCA 5 has a defect on chromosome 15. The SCA 2 is common in India, and has slow pursuit eye movements. On asking the patient to move the eyes to the right or left, he initiates the movements with a jerk of the head, the eyes following subsequently. They may also have mild mental retardation and bilateral ptosis. Optic atrophy is rare while signs of pyramidal involvement are generally present. Proprioceptive deficits, peripheral neuropathy and extra-pyramidal signs may be present in varying combinations. Kyphoscoliosis is present, but pes cavus is usually not seen. The defect in SCA 8 is on chromosome 13q21, and has cerebellar atrophy with pyramidal signs and cognitive impairment. On the other hand the SCA10 is due to ATTCT pentanucleotide repeat on chromosome 22q13 and have ataxia with seizures. SCA 14 is a late onset, slowly progressive ataxia with genetic defect on chromosome 19q 13qter while SCA 16 has the genetic defect on chromosome 8q 22.1-24.1.

DENTATO-RUBRAL PALLIDO LUYSIAN ATROPHY (DRPLA) is another form of dominant ataxia. It has a wide range at age at onset. The syndrome is again a triplet repeat disease with genetic defect on chromosome 12. The ataxia is associated with choreoathetosis, myoclonus, epilepsy and dementia.

THE SEX-LINKED VARIETY has signs of cerebellar degeneration, with slowly progressive muscle atrophy, pyramidal weakness and brisk reflexes with extensor plantar response. There may be position and vibration sense lost. The spinal cord pathology is like Friedreich's ataxia. Pes cavus, scoliosis and increased lumbar lordosis are associated. The other sex-linked variety with a defective gene at xq13, is associated with sideroblastic anaemia and has phospho-glycerokinase as the metabolic defect.

ATAXIA TELENGIECTASIA is a progressive disorder that affects the cerebellum, in the first or second decade of life. Telengectasia of the conjunctivae and tendency to recurrent infections due to hypo or agamma-globulinemia are other notable features of this disease. The patient dies of intercurrent infection.

Ataxia can occur due to cerebellar haemorrhage and may sometimes present as an emergency. A severe occipital headache, vomiting and ataxia herald the onset of this catastrophic illness. If deterioration in consciousness is noted the haematoma has to be evacuated as an emergency. CAT scan establishes the diagnosis. Cerebellar abscess, granulomas and cerebellar tumours also present with slowly progressive ataxia and signs of increased intracranial tension. For tuberculomas, AKT can be tried initially, and appropriate antibiotics should be tried for other types of granulomas. Surgery when indicated should be offered for all the lesions.

In a wide variety of diseases, a combination of ataxia and other neurological abnormalities exists. Following list is useful in the differential diagnosis

Table 4.1

Ataxia Plus Syndromes

ATAXIA+MENTAL RETARDATION	Ataxic cerebral palsy, congenital ataxias, early onset recessive ataxias, Xeroderma pigmentosum
ATXIA + DEMENTIA	Degenerative(SCA, Ataxia telangiectasia, Myoclonic epilepsy) Metabolic (Metachromatic leukodystrophy, adrenoleukodystrophy, Wilson's disease, Dystonic lipidosis, hypothyroidism) Toxic (heavy metal, Phenytoin) Infection (CJD, SSPE) Neoplastic
ATAXIA+OPTIC ATROPHY	Multiple sclerosis, Freidreich's ataxia, inherited ataxias
ATAXIA+RETINOPATHY	Inherited ataxias, Mitochondrial disorders
ATAXIA+EXTRAPYRAMIDAL SIGNS	Wilson's disease, Ataxia telangiectasia, Dominant late onset ataxia
ATAXIA+SUPRANUCLEAR OPTHALMOPLEGIA	Dominant ataxias, OPCA, idiopathic late onset ataxias, Hexosaminidase deficiency, Niemenn Pick disease

SENSORY SYSTEM

Anatomists divide the sensations into somatic and visceral. Most of the sensations tested clinically fall into somatic group. Somatosensory system is concerned with perceptions of body sensations from skin surface, joints and muscles.

Two kinds of somatic sensations are clinically tested.

1. Exteroceptive : Includes pain, temperature and tactile sensations.
2. Proprioceptive: Includes sense of position, sense of vibration, pressure and deep pain sensation.

   If above two modalities are relatively intact, then we also check

3. Cortical sensations: which include two-point discrimination, tactile extinction, stereognosis, graphesthesia, tactile localisation.

ANATOMY OF SOMATO SENSORY SYSTEM:

There are two major components of somatosensory system for the body and only one for the head. The two components for the body are the dorsal column or medial leminiscus system and the spinothalamic or spinal leminiscus system. The trigeminal system is for the head.

DORSAL COLUMN OR MEDIAL LEMINISCUS SYSTEM:

Large myelinated fibres arising from encapsulated nerve endings form these tracts and carry proprioception — the position and vibration senses along with crude touch. Information from the receptor is carried to the neuraxis by distal and the proximal processes of ganglion cells, the bipolar neurones which constitute the first order neurons. The proximal processes of ganglion cells enter the spinal cord via dorsal roots and ascend in posterior funiculus as fasciculus gracilis (column of Goll). They carry proprioceptive sensations from sacral, lumbar and lower thoracic dermatomes. Fasciculus cuneatus (column of Burdach) lying laterally to fasciculus gracilis carries sensations from upper thoracic and cervical areas. The second order fibres arising from nucleus gracilis and cuneatus decussate in lower medulla (sensory decussation) and ascend in the brainstem as medial leminiscus, and relay into third order neurons of thalamus and ultimately to post rolandic cortex.

SPINOTHALAMIC OR SPINAL LEMINISCUS SYSTEM

These tracts are formed by small unmyelinated fibres arising from free nerve endings and carry pain, temperature and fine touch which is less discriminative. First order neurons are situated in the dorsal root ganglia. Distal processes bring the information from free nerve endings, and proximal processes relay in the substantia gelatinosa after ascending or descending a few segments. The substantia gelatinosa is located within the grey matter of dorsal horn of spinal cord and the fibres arising from it, cross the midline in anterior commisure. After crossing, these fibres form ventral and lateral spino-thalamic tracts. The fibres are arranged in the spino-thalamic tract in an orderly manner called the lamination. The fibres from lower parts of body are located postero-laterally and those from upper parts are situated antero-laterally. This lamination forms the basis of various pattern of sensory impairment in cord lesions. Also, temperature fibres are more towards the midline than pain fibres. At the junction of spinal cord and the medulla, the spino-thalamic tract turns into spinal lemniscus and which relays to ventro-postero-lateral thalamic nucleus and then to the somato sensory cortex.

There is a descending system from cortex via periaqueductal nuclei, relaying into substantia gelatinosa, which can modulate the pain perception. It is of note that tactile sensation carried by dorsal column is concerned with accurate localisation and discrimination while that carried by spino-thalamic tract lacks accurate localisation. Due to overlap between the two systems, tactile sensations are least affected with spinal cord lesions.

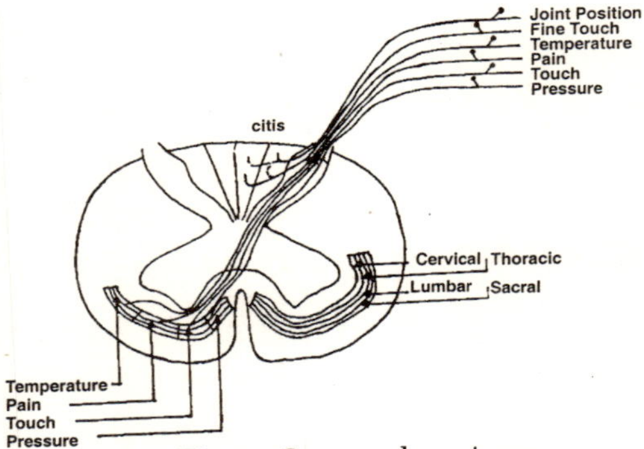

Fig 4.1 Sensory lemniscus

TRIGEMINAL SYSTEM: is fully discussed in Chapter II under the Vth nerve.

SOMATO-SENSORY CORTEX

The somato-sensory cortex is located in the post central gyrus and subserves the sensations from the contralateral side of the body in the 'homunculus' i.e. somatotropic arrangement of body in inverted order with lower limb superiorly located to face and upper limbs. Maximum representation is devoted to those areas of body where somatic sensations are most vital.

Somatosensory cortex is concerned with the discriminative and higher aspects of sensations like stereognosis and graphesthesia. Conscious awareness of pain is achieved at thalamic level but the discriminative aspects are appreciated at cortical level.

SENSORY DERMATOMES

Dermatome is an area on skin supplied by a particular spinal segment. Figures 4.2 and 4.3 show the distribution of sensory dermatomes. Patient should be considered as standing with palms of hands facing forwards. Some important points to remember are as follows. C_1 does not supply the skin, C_5 supplies outer aspect of shoulder tip, T_3 lies in the axilla, T_8, T_{10}, T_{12} supply rib margin, umbilicus and pubis respectively, L_3 lies at the knees, L_5 is at outer aspect of leg to inner foot, S_1 is at outer aspect of foot including the little toe and S_3, S_4, S_5 lie concentrically around anus.

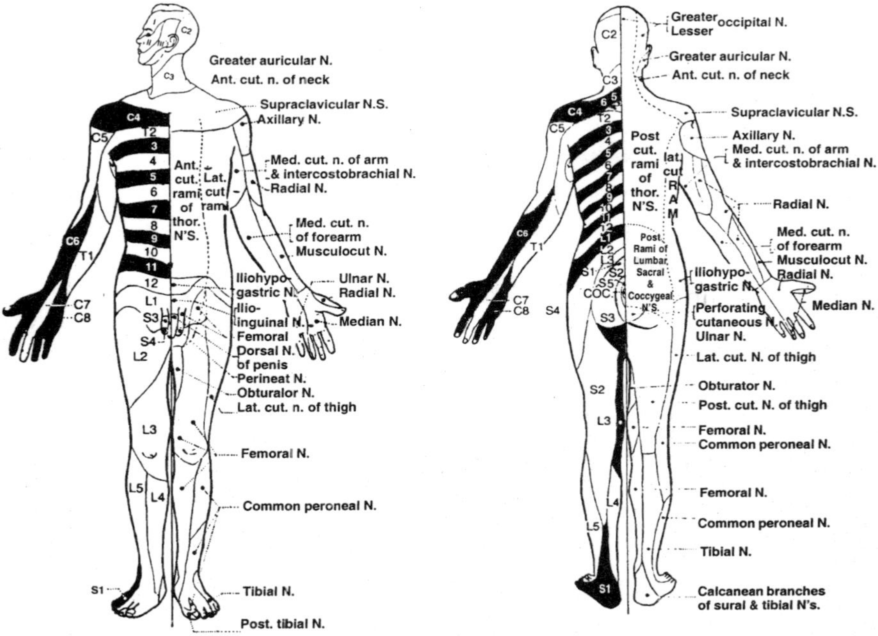

Figs 4.2 and 4.3 Sensory dermatomes on right and the nerve supply on the left

CLINICAL EXAMINATION:

Sensory examination is one of the most difficult parts of the clinical neurological examination. Patient's co-operation is of utmost importance. When the history points to the involvement of the sensory system, it is worthwhile examining the sensations before the patient or the examiner begins to get distracted.

PAIN: Gently touch with a sharp pin on the skin surface, which is expected to be normal from the history and let the patient feel the sharpness. Then delineate the areas of decreased sensation moving from impaired towards normal sensations, as the change to normal is easier to appreciate. Start from distal areas and move proximally.

TEMPERATURE: Use a test tube with hot water having temperature around 43 degrees centigrade for the sensation of heat and a test tube with ice less than 30 degrees centigrade for testing the cold sensation. The cold test tube should be kept dry. Avoid extremes of hot and cold sensations as they stimulate pain fibres rather than temperature.

TOUCH: A small wisp of cotton or the examiner's finger is best for testing tactile sensation. Patient is asked whether he feels the touch and whether it is different from the feeling at other areas.

JOINT POSITION: (proprioception): A distal joint is moved and with the patients eyes closed and he is told to inform the direction of movements. Take care not to put pressure on the nail. If impaired, proceed to test the proximal joints.

VIBRATION SENSE: A tuning fork vibrating at 128 Hz is placed over a distal bony prominence (e.g. medial malleolus) and patient is asked to report whether he feels the vibrations. It is important that his eyes are closed. If he says that he can feel the vibrations, then the fork is stopped from vibrating and patient is asked whether vibrations are still present, in order to check that he/she is not guessing. If impaired, proceed to proximal bony prominences.

TWO POINT DISCRIMINATION: Two pinheads (and not the sharp ends) are simultaneously placed at pulp of fingers and patient is expected to perceive both of them. On finger pulp it is possible to discriminate up to less than 5mm distance but over dorsum of foot, 5 cm may be the minimum separation needed to perceive the two stimuli individually.

GRAPHESTHESIA: Patient is asked to report the exact figure of the digit traced by the examiner on the palm, hand or foot with eyes closed.

STEREOGNOSIS: Patient is asked to identify the object placed in his palm, by its texture and form with eyes closed.

TACTILE LOCALISATION: Is checked by asking the patient to precisely locate the area touched by the examiner.

Table 4.2

Common Definitions:

Anaesthesia:	Loss of all modalities of sensation
Hypaesthesia	Partial loss of almost all modalities
Analgesia	Loss of pain
Hypalgesia	Partial loss of pain
Allodynia	Spontaneous abnormal sensations like burning, tingling
Dysesthesia	Spontaneous painful sensations.

VARIOUS PATTERNS OF SENSORY IMPAIRMENT

1. UNILATERAL LOSS OF ALL MODALITIES of sensations is seen with contralateral thalamic lesion. Usual aetiology is cerebral vascular disease. Hysterical patients may also complain of similar impairment.

2. IMPAIRED PAIN AND TEMPERATURE on one side with facial sensations impaired on other side is seen with brain stem lesion involving the ascending spino-thalamic and descending spinal tract of Vth nerve. e.g. lateral medullary syndrome (Wallenburg's Syndrome).

3. IMPAIRMENT OF ALL MODALITIES OF SENSATIONS below a definite level over the body is seen with spinal cord pathologies like acute transverse myelitis. Note that the level over the skin surface does not correspond to the vertebral level. Often there is a zone of hyperaesthesia overlying the sensory level.

4. BROWN-SEQUARD SYNDROME indicates that the lesion is likely to be below the level of foramen magnum and is often the result of extramedullary compression, although intramedullary lesions like traumatic gun shot injuries to one side of cord can also rarely produce the syndrome.

5. SUSPENDED SENSORY IMPAIRMENT AND DISSOCIATED SENSORY LOSS:. Intramedullary lesions like syringomyelia lead

to involvement of central portions of the spinal cord. Here the spino-thalamic fibres, crossing in the anterior commissure are affected and cause a sensory loss of pain and temperature over the involved dermatomes. Sensation carried in the posterior column is spared as the posterior columns are away from the central portions of the cord. This is the dissociated sensory loss. The dissociated sensory loss extends for a few segments, above and below these segments, the sensations are normal. This is called the suspended sensory loss. Sacral sensations are intact, as the fibres are situated most laterally in the cord.

6. 'SADDLE' ANAESTHESIA. Impairment of sensation over the buttock area (i.e. saddle) is seen with tumours of conus medullaris, like ependymoma.

7. SENSORY ATAXIA: Involvement of posterior columns carrying the proprioception leads to sensory ataxia. The patient is unaware of the exact position of the limbs and it worsens markedly with the suppression of visual cues i.e. eyes closed (Romberg's sign). Typically, subacute combined degeneration is responsible for sensory ataxia and must be diagnosed, as it is treatable. Arnold Chiari malformation and Friedreich's ataxia can also lead to sensory ataxia. In older days tabes dorsalis used to be very common cause of sensory ataxia but is not frequently seen these days.

8. GLOVE AND STOCKING HYPOAESTHESIA: Peripheral loss of sensation involving distal feet and hand is a feature of peripheral neuropathy.

9. LOSS OF ALL MODALITIES OF SENSATIONS over a clearly defined area is one part of the body only could be due to a lesion of a sensory root or peripheral nerve. Noting the pattern of sensory impairment can give the clue between these two sites of lesion. Common causes of mono neuropathies are Hansen's disease, vasculitis, entrapment neuropathies (e.g. carpal tunnel syndrome) and diabetes.

Table 4.3

Causes Of Sensory Ataxia

Vitamin B12 deficiency
Tabes Dorsalis
Freidreich's Ataxia
Diabetic neuropathy
Hereditary Sensory Motor Neuropathy
Hereditary Sensory Neuropathy
Vitanmin E deficiency
HIV related Vacuolar Myelopathy
Ganglionopathies
Cranio-vertebral Junction anomalies

SYRINGOMYELIA:

The word syrinx means a rock cut tunnel and myelia means spinal cord. Syringomyelia is defined as a cavity in the substance of spinal cord which could be either communicating or non-communicating depending upon its communication with the central canal. It is usually due to abnormalities at cranio vertebral junction obstructing the outflow of CSF from the fourth ventricle through foramen of Lushka and Magendie and thus pressure waves get transmitted down the central canal through which syrinx develops as an out pouching. Arnold Chiari malformation (downward herniation of cerebellar tonsil through foramen magnum) is commonly associated with syringomyelia. Syrinx can also be associated with spinal cord tumours or can be a sequel of spinal cord trauma or arachnoiditis.

Clinically, patient develops cape like suspended sensory impairment over the chest (as cervical and upper dorsal cord is the commonest site for syrinx), along with wasting and weakness of both upper extremities (lower motor neurone involvement). Often painless ulcers develop over fingers. Horner's syndrome due to involvement of sympathetic tracts is commonly noted. Lower limbs show spasticity and if the syrinx extends into the lower brainstem (syringobulbia) dysphagia, dysarthria and lower cranial nerve dysfunction develop. The disease is very slowly progressive. Diagnosis is made by cervical cord MRI that shows the syrinx, and associated spinal cord tumour. If present the treatment suggested is surgical removal of the tumour. However, no consensus is yet available, as the natural course of the disease is unpredictable. If the syrinx is progressive surgical drainage may also be considered. Various types of surgical procedures have been advocated such as section of the filum terminale etc.

SUBACUTE COMBINED DEGENERATION:

The disease is subacute in onset, with degeneration of dorsal columns and cortico-spinal tracts. The condition is due to deficiency of vitamin B_{12} due to lack of intrinsic factor with achlorhydria (pernicious anaemia). Vitamin B_{12} deficiency may also occur due to dietary deficiency (common in India) or its malabsorbtion due to coeliac disease, tropical sprue, intestinal tuberculosis, regional ileitis, and diverticulosis or total/partial gastrectomy. Full-blown clinical picture of Vitamin B_{12} deficiency consists of macrocytic anaemia, atrophic glossitis and neurological complications. Latter includes subacute progressive, spastic with sensory ataxic syndrome with peripheral neuropathy (bilateral ankle jerks are absent). Romberg's sign is positive. Often optic atrophy and cognitive decline are associated. Demonstrating a low Vitamin B_{12} level (< 170 pg/ml) establishes the diagnosis. Elevated serum methylmalonic acid and homocysteinic levels are also present and can be used for diagnosis. If Vitamin. B_{12} levels are abnormal, treatment is by supplementation of Vitamin. B_{12} The treatment consists of parenteral vitamin B_{12} in the doses of 1000 micrograms daily for 15 days followed by a maintenance dose of 1000 microgram per month. The prognosis is very good if treatment is started early.

CHAPTER V

INFECTIONS OF THE NERVOUS SYSTEM

Infection may reach the central nervous system via multiple routes. It may result from direct spread as in osteomyelitis of the skull or vertebrae, mastoiditis or sinusitis. Infection may come via the blood stream (haematogenous) or spread along the anastamotic veins that connect the facial and intracranial venous channels. Penetrating brain wounds can introduce infection and lastly infection may be introduced iatrogenically during a lumbar puncture using unsterile equipment, or during surgery. The iatrogenic causes of infections are fortunately very rare.

A variety of organisms can cause infection of the nervous system:

BACTERIA: Meningococci, Pneumococci, Pneumocystis carinii, Streptococci, Haemophilus influenzae, Listeria monocytogenis and Mycobacterium tuberculosis are the commonest bacterial infections of the nervous system. Listeria monocytogenis infection occurs during old age, or with diabetes, ethanol abuse or due to immuno-compromisation. Children and young adults are usually infected by Meningococci or N. meningitides. The nerves, both cranial and peripheral may get infected with mycobacterium leprae. Rarely staphylococcus gains entry via catheters and shunts introduced in the brain or spinal canal, or following Neurosurgery, head trauma and endocarditis. S. Pseudomonas and flavobacteria infect the nervous tissue during assisted ventilation. Infection with Gram negative bacilli occurs after trauma, neurosurgery, ruptured brain abscess, or following systemic infection in sickle cell disease, cirrhosis or myeloma. Patients with HIV infection and AIDS, or on immunosuppressive drugs and patients with carcinoma are more likely to fall prey to infections with Gram negative organisms and rare organisms such as Toxoplasma gondii. Whipple's disease caused by bacteria called Trophenryma whippelii is occasionally seen in India.

VIRUSES: Common viruses infecting the central nervous system are Entero viruses like Echo virus, Coxsackie virus, Polio virus, Influenza virus A and B. Meningoencephalitis complicating infectious fevers due to illnesses like measles, mumps and the variola-zoster group of viruses. The other viruses are Epstein-Barr virus, Herpes simplex and retroviruses like human T cell lymphotropic virus type 1and HIV 1 and 2.

SPIROCHETES: Treponema pallidum (Syphilis), Leptospira interogenus and Borrelia burgdorferi.

FUNGI AND YEAST: The fungi that infect the CNS and rarely spinal cord are: Cryptococci, Coccidioides, Candida, Histoplasma Capsulatum, Actinomycetes, Aspergilosis, Blastomycosis, Mucormycosis and Torula.

PARASITES: Malaria, Cysticercosis, Amoebiasis and Trypanosomiasis, Toxoplasma gondii, Schistosoma and Angiostrongylus.

Inflammation can also occur due to exposure to chemical agents and after infiltration by malignant cells.

When an inflammatory process involves the pia and arachnoid membranes the resultant condition is called *leptomeningitis,* where as inflammation of the dura alone is called *pachymeningitis.* The term meningitis is generally used to mean leptomeningeal involvement.

MENINGITIS

The leptomeninges may be infected by any of the agents listed above. However, certain organisms are commoner in specific age groups. In neonates below one month of age, E. Coli or Group B streptococcus infection is common while in infants up to 2 years of age, infection with S.pneumoniae, N.meningitides or Group B streptococcus is common. In adolescence N.meningitides, S.pneumoniae, H.Influenzae or Group B streptococcus infection is known to cause meningitis. While in adults and elderly S. pneumoniae, N.meningitides, L. monocytogenes, Group B Streptococcus or H. Influenzae are the likely organisms causing meningitis.

In neonates, the mortality and morbidity is high after an attack of meningitis. Almost 50% succumb to meningitis. Despite improvement in antibiotic therapy, the morbidity has also not improved specially in the domains of learning and neuromotor functions.

PATHOGENESIS OF SEPTIC MENINGITIS : Bacteria have to gain access in the CSF to cause meningeal infection and inflammation. To do so, they have to travel through the blood brain barrier or have a direct access to CSF following surgery, or penetrating injuries. Usually the bacteria colonise in the nasopharyngeal mucosal epithelium. In the nasopharynx bacteria secrete IgA proteases to neutralise the action of plasma cell mediated mucosal IgA. They then invade the adjacent intravascular space, but before doing so, they have to survive the initial complement mediated defences of the host. The bacterial capsule made of polysaccharide helps the bacteria evade the action of serum complement. The bacteria have outer adhesive pili, which help them to attach themselves to the nasopharyngeal mucosa and vascular endothelium. They then translocate through the endothelial gap and enter the CSF where they finally survive and replicate. The chances of survival are more as the initial host response generates minimal immunoglobulins and complement mediated humoral defences. It is said that initially there is only 50 % opsonic activity, which increases as the infection persists and the defence mechanism upgrades.

NISSERIA MENINGITIDES (MENINGOCOCCAL) MENINGITIS: N.meningitides is a Gram-negative encapsulated bacillus occurring in pairs. The incidence of meningococcal meningitis is highest in infants and very young children (1-23 months) but no age is a bar. It forms 25 % of all bacterial meningitis. It is said to be commoner in the early months of the year. Infection reaches the nervous system via the nasopharynx and is transmitted by human contacts. There is no maternal to foetal transmission. A septicaemia heralds the onset of the disease. There is high fever, malaise, and severe headache. Purpuric rash and the Waterhouse-Friedrichsen syndrome, which results from haemorrhage in the adrenal glands following disseminated intravascular coagulopathy, may occur during this stage. Intense headache, restlessness, irritability, delirium and seizures herald meningitis. Herpetic eruption may be seen around the mouth. Metastatic infection involving the eyes – uveitis and choroiditis, the bones – purulent arthritis, the heart – myocarditis may complicate the course of the illness. The temperature is elevated, ranging from 39 to 40 degrees centigrade. Marked stiffness of the neck, and a positive Kernig's and Brudzinski signs are found on examination. In the initial stages, there are no focal neurological signs, but the reflexes may be exaggerated. Adhesions of the leptomeninges may obstruct the CSF pathway leading to hydrocephalus. The optic and auditory nerves may be severely damaged as a result of infection. Chronic meningococcal septicaemia may also be complicated by a meningeal infection. Purpura, arthritis and low-grade fever accompany the condition that results from a deficiency of the IgM immunoglobulin complex. Cutaneous scars, amputations due to purulent arthritis and renal injury are other common complications.

Meningococcal meningitis can be differentiated from other forms of meningitis by the isolation of meningococci from CSF. Pneumococcal meningitis is diagnosed by demonstrating pneumococci in the CSF. Gram-negative bacilli are seen in Haemophilus infection. The CSF shows similar findings in all types of purulent meningitis. The opening pressure is elevated above 180 mm of mercury; the fluid is turbid and has a polymorphonuclear pleocytosis around 1,00 to 20,000 cells. Protein content is markedly increased around 100 – 500 mg/dl, whilst glucose is decreased below 40 mg/dl and may even be zero. The CSF chloride level depends on the serum chloride and is lowered if there has been persisting vomiting.

Meningococcal meningitis is treated by the use of benzyl or crystalline penicillin in a dose of 50,000 units/kg intravenously in six divided doses. In adults the dose of penicillin is 24 to 30 mega units per day in four to six divided doses. About 4 % of strains are resistant to penicillin. Ceftriaxone in children is given in a dose of 75mgm/kg every 8 hours and 2 G. every 8 hours to adults. Cefotaxime is used in children in a dose of 50-75/mg/kg every 6 hours and 2 G every 6 hours in adults. Chloramphenicol is used for patients, who are allergic to penicillin, in a dose of 25 mg/kg/day in four divided doses for children and in a dose of one gram 6 hourly for adults. It is important to treat the household contacts with chemoprophylaxis, as approximately 4 cases out of every thousand contacts develop meningitis. Rifampicin is given in the dose of 600 mg twice a day for 2 days for adults and for infants younger than one month old in the dose of 5mg/kg and for older children 10 mg/kg. The contact lenses may become discoloured due to it. It is contraindicated in pregnancy. Ciprofloxacin or oral Azithromycin is also useful in a single dose of 500 mg, but it is not recommended for persons under 18 years of age and in pregnant and lactating women. For pregnant women intramuscular Ceftriaxone is recommended in a single dose of 250 mg. Vaccines are under trial.

S.PNEUMONIAE are gram-positive cocci occurring in pairs. They have an external capsule, which protect them from phagocytosis by the host's polymorphonuclear cells. For pneumococci, the nasopharynx is the site for colonisation in 10 % of adults and 40 % of children. Infection can also occur from nasal sinuses or middle ear. It also spreads from person to person by respiratory droplets, in crowded places like cinema halls, theatres, barracks, day care centres and prisons. Nosoconial spread is also known. In adults, diabetes, liver disease, alcohol, HIV infection or splenectomy are the predisposing factors. Initially pneumococcal pneumonia may occur.

The symptoms are similar to meningococcal meningitis. Penicillin is the treatment of choice. In infection with penicillin resistant strain, 3rd generation cephalosporins, such as Cefotaxime or Ceftriaxone or newer fluoroquinolones such as Levofloxacin or Sparfloxacin are recommended. Combination of Vancomycin with Ceftriaxone is better than either of them alone. It must be remembered that penetration of Vancomycin in the CSF is diminished in the presence of dexamethasone and hence the combination. Vancomycin is given in the dose of 15/kg every 6 hours in children and 1 G every 12 hours in adults. The dose of Cefotaxime is 50-75 mg/kg every 6 hours in children and 2 G, 6 hourly in adults. Ceftraixone is used in the dose of 75 mg/kg every 8 hours in children and 2G every 8 hours in adults. The third generation cephalosporins can be combined with Rifampicin and dexamethasone does not alter the levels of either . The dose of Rifampicin is 10 mg/kg every 24 hours in children and 600 mg every 24 hours in adults. The fatality rate is around 20 %.

Meningitis due to GROUP B STREPTOCOCCUS occurs in infants due to intrapartum transmission from mother's genital tracts. It is more common in premature children with low birth weight. Nosoconial spread occurs in almost 25% of cases. Combination of Penicillin with Ampicillin and Gentamycin is the treatment of choice. The dose of Gentamycin is 2.5 mg/kg every 8 hours in children and 2mg/kg as a loading dose followed by 1.7 mg/kg every 8 hours in adults.

The incidence of H. INFLUENZAE meningitis has been reduced after the introduction of vaccine for both types A and B. It is a gram negative, small cocco bacillus with an outer capsule. There is no natural host and is transferred from person to person. The case fatality is around 5 %. Resistance to Ceftriaxone and Cefotaxime is not seen. Prevention is by administration of Rifampicin in the dose of 20mg/kg (600-mg maximum) in a single daily dose before breakfast for 4 days. The vaccine should be administered to all, the first dose being given at 23 months of age.

L. MONOCYTOGENUS BETA HAEMOLYTICUS are gram negative, anaerobic rods. It infects elderly, diabetics, people with ethanol abuse and/or immunocompromised. After phagocytosis, the organisms cause lysis of the phagocytosome and escape into the cytoplasm of the cell where it proliferates. It then migrates to the periphery of the cell causing a protrusion and is ingested by the adjoining cell. Which ultimately sets the infective cycle into motion. Organisms enter the blood stream either through leucocytes or as free organisms after cell lysis. The organisms are food borne and usually found in Cole slaw, pasteurised milk or soft cheese. Combination of Penicillin, Ampicillin and Gentamycin is the treatment of choice. In rare circumstance when the organism is resistant to penicillin Trimethoprim with Sulfamethoxone is used. Bacterial meningitis even today, has large morbidity and mortality. Introduction of vaccines for each organism causing serious meningitis may help to lower the incidence of meningitis.

RECURRENT MENINGITIS can occur due to anatomical defects, which are congenital, post-operative or traumatic. It also occurs in auto-immune diseases and immunodeficiency states. The idiopathic variety is known as Mollaret's meningitis. With every recurrent episode, symptoms like acute bacterial meningitis develop, however, the constitutional symptoms are less. The CSF shows large fragile cells resembling endothelial cells, which are probably monocytes. Based on PCR HSV-2 is implicated. Rare cases are due to HSV-1 or Epstein Barr viral infection.

TUBERCULAR MENINGITIS: This particular meningeal infection is rampant throughout India and may account for 5 to 8 % of all infections occurring in the country.

Mycobacterium bovis, Africanus and avian (usually with AIDS) can cause disease in humans but mycobacterium tuberculosis is the commonest cause of central nervous system (CNS) infection. It is an obligate aerobic organism. It is non-motile and non-spore forming and has a slow growth. The cell division occurs every 20 to 24 hours; hence the infection has a chronic course. The entire mycobacterial genome is now sequenced. It has a circular chromosome and is the largest genome among the bacteria. It has all the enzymes, capable of synthesising all the essential nutrients including lipids and glycolipids. It is now getting recognised that the mycobacterium can have a system for antigenic variation.

The granulomatous nodular lesions in the lungs provide less number of bacteria than the cavitating lesions. The severity of these lesions determines the individual's capacity to be contagious. It is transmitted from person to person by inhalation of aerosolised droplet nuclei. The mycobacterium so inhaled, multiply in the alveolar spaces or macrophages. They are killed within 2 to 4 weeks. Some survive and spread via haematogenous route to all extrapulmonary sites including the CNS. MRI has shown presence of asymptomatic granulomas in CNS during the course of milliary tuberculosis. These granulomas are tubercles consisting of necrotic caseous centre surrounded by mononuclear cells. They are seen in lungs and extrapulmonary sites including CNS. In the CNS it has been called Rich focus, which develops early in the course of infection. The location of this expanding focus determines the type of CNS infection one is likely to encounter in a given patient. This focus rupturing in the subarachnoid space causes meningitis. Deeper in the brain and spinal cord, conglomeration and expansion produces space occupying tuberculomas or abscess. The abscess is rare.

Tuberculosis can affect the CNS in several ways, as meningitis, as tuberculomas in the brain and spinal cord parenchyma, as infection of the vertebrae (Pott's spine) which may lead to compression of the cord and paraplegia and finally chronically as arachnoiditis.

In early meningitis a diffuse exudate made up of neutrophils, mononuclear cells, erythrocytes and viable tubercle bacilli within a loose fibrin network is found in the basal subarachnoid space. At the base of the brain, the cranial nerves are at times surrounded by this exudate. The infection is also found around the choroid plexus. As disease progresses, lymphocytes and connective tissue elements tend to predominate in the subarachnoid space. Small and medium size blood vessels passing through the exudates become inflamed giving rise to vasculitis. The thrombosis of these inflamed vessels can lead to infarction of the brain parenchyma. Further, the brain parenchyma adjacent to the exudate gets damaged leading to border zone encephalitis.

Protein purified derivative (PPD) reactivity develops and provides together with the radiological changes, indications for infection.

Tubercular meningitis can occur at any age though it is commoner in children. Tubercular meningitis usually occurs following tuberculosis elsewhere in the body. In the prodormal period, the non-specific symptoms like fatigue, malaise, myalgia and low evening rise of temperature are common. The British Medical Research council has advocated a staging system.

Stage 1: Patient fully conscious, rational, and with no neurological signs, has systemic symptoms and signs of meningeal irritation.

Stage 2: Patient confused, but not comatose with hemiparesis and single cranial nerve palsy, mainly 6th nerve in over 25 % of patients.

Stage 3: Patient comatose or stuperose, multiple cranial nerve palsies – usually 3rd, 4th, 7th and 8th, with complete hemiplegia or paraplegia.

In the first stage of meningitis, a vague history of illness, with infection of the upper respiratory tract and apathy is reported.

Irritability, lack of appetite, and low-grade fever with lethargy out of proportion to other symptoms, are the classical symptoms, which are often missed or ascribed to other causes. Mild to moderate hyponatremia may be encountered in over 50 % of patients, due to syndrome of inappropriate antidiuretic hormone secretion (SIADH). The chest radiograph may be positive for tubercular infection, with positive tuberculin test, more often in adults and meningeal inflammation is noted on scanning with contrast administration. Choroidal tubercles are seen in 10 % of cases with milliary tuberculosis. Extra CNS tuberculosis like pulmonary lesions, lymph node enlargement or spinal tuberculosis is noted in about 60 % of cases with meningitis.

In over 50 % of cases the onset is acute, the patient presenting with fever, headache, vomiting and having had several seizures. In adults the onset may be subacute, with a history of confusion, loss of memory etc., and focal signs such as mono or hemi paresis. Rarely, a child is brought to the hospital in coma with signs of acute hydrocephalus and rapid deterioration. If diagnosis is missed in the early stages, irregular remittent fever, drowsiness, irritability and confusion occur.

It is interesting to note that pulmonary tuberculosis and/or lymphadenopathy occurs more commonly in Tubercular meningitis with AIDS – 50 % versus 3 % in non-HIV patients. Secondly, 16 % of patients with AIDS have acellular CSF initially, as compared to 3 % in patients without AIDS. The cells rise in 24 - 48 hours.

The CSF shows a lymphocytic pleocytosis and glucose levels, which though lower than normal, is not as low as in purulent meningitis. Very early cases of tubercular meningitis may show a polymorphonuclear preponderance, and may be mistaken for purulent meningitis. The routine CSF examination helps to reach the diagnosis. Demonstration of tubercle bacilli on smear, culture, PCR or after guinea pig inoculation confirms the clinical suspicion. Though not specific, CSF adenosine deaminase levels are raised in 90 % of tubercular meningitis cases. They are also raised in other conditions like lymphoma with meningeal involvement, subarachnoid haemorrhage and sarcoidosis. False negative test is also seen. Cut-off value is between 5 & 10 IU/l. Sensitivity and specificity is high in adults though elevated levels can be seen with bacterial, viral and tubercular meningitis in children. The level is raised in the first two weeks before therapy and that once treatment is started it progressively diminishes. For demonstration of bacilli, PCR is more sensitive as compared to microscopic examination and culture. Patients with atypical history or with focal neurological signs or cranial nerve palsies may need further investigations like CAT scan and MRI imaging with contrast administration. The imaging techniques show enhancement of basal cisterns, interpeduncular fossa, ambient cisterns and chiasmatic regions, in post contrast CAT and MRI scans. Obstructive hydrocephalus and/or cerebral atrophy may be demonstrated, the latter being more common in patients with coexistent HIV infection. One may also demonstrate narrowing of the arteries at the base or occluded small vessels with basal ganglia or cortical infarcts. Arteritis may also be demonstrated on MR angiography or digital subtraction angiography (DSA).

The course of the disease is radically altered by the prompt administration of antitubercular therapy. However, mortality and morbidity is more in patients with associated HIV infection. Treatment consists of the administration of three or four antitubercular drugs at the onset. The first line drugs are injection Streptomycin, Isoniazide, Rifampicin, Ethambutol and Pyrizinamide. If no response is obtained or if the bacilli are resistant to these drugs, the second line drugs are, Para-aminosalicylic acid (PAS), Ethionamide, Cycloserine, some aminoglycosides like Kanamycin and quinolones. Rifabutin is used in patients with AIDS, instead of Rifampicin as the latter drug has interaction with antiretroviral therapy. Intramuscularly Streptomycin is administered in the dose of 40 mg/kg in children and 1 to 2 grams in adults, together with Isoniazide, 5mg/kg in children and 300-400 mg/day in adults, for patients less than 50kg. body weight, Rifampicin is usually given on an empty stomach in a single dose of 450 mg in adults below 50kg in weight and in the dose of 600 mg in persons over 50kg body weight. Children usually receive 10-20mg/kg. Ethambutol is used in the dosage of 15 – 25 mg/kg, while Pyrazinamide is used in the dose of 1.5G. in adults below 50kg body weight, 2G for persons above 50kg and 2.5G for patients above 75kg while children are administered a dose of 40mg/kg/day. Thiacetazone to adults is given in the dose of

50mg/kg/day while to children in the dose of 40mg/kg/day. The old drug Paraaminosalycylic is used in the dose 10-15g/day. The dose of Ethionamide is 0.75g/day in adults below 50kg in weight and 1G/ day in adults over 50kg.

Steroids are generally administered simultaneously as they help to reduce inflammation and the risk of adhesions, and also improve the general state of the patient especially in terms of a feeling of well-being and an increased appetite. Their role in initial stages of the disease is controversial. All drugs should be continued for a period of three months and CSF examination carried out every 2-3 weeks to monitor the progress of the disease. If a satisfactory response is not observed in the first 3 weeks, the diagnosis should be doubted, or the presence of AIDS or complications suspected. A rise in CSF protein levels should lead to a suspicion of adhesive arachnoiditis and hydrocephalus, which are usually associated with the chronicity of the illness. MRI examination will help the diagnosis and to delineate the extent of the lesion. A ventriculo-peritoneal shunt may have to be inserted otherwise the patient may lapse into coma. The use of intrathecal Hyalurinidase (1500 units) every 15 days has been suggested to treat adhesions especially in the spinal form of the disease.

Spinal arachnoiditis can be one of the common complication of, or the only manifestation of, tubercular meningitis. It may present subacutely or in a chronic form. The subacute form begins with radicular pains that resemble the pain of sciatica. The pains tend to involve multiple roots. The root involvement gradually ascends, and the pain radiates down the arms. Pain varies from a dull ache to a lancinating character. As the spinal cord may also be involved, a spastic paraplegia or quadriplegia may be seen. Due to root and cord involvement a mixed type of paralysis is seen in the upper limbs. There is wasting and weakness of the small muscles of the hands. Fasciculation may be observed in the deltoids, biceps and the flexors of the forearms. There is inversion of the supinator reflex, the reflex itself being absent, with exaggeration of finger flexion. Sphincter involvement occurs early in the course of the disease. Paraesthesia and dysesthesias are common starting at the sacral level and ascending to the trunk. On examination there is proprioceptive loss in the lower limbs.

The CSF is xanthochromic with a lymphocytic pleocytosis, and a marked increase in protein. The glucose is low in tubercular variety of arachnoiditis. Syphilis can cause a similar symptom complex and is diagnosed by positive VDRL reaction and Wasserman test in the CSF. CAT scan and MRI with gadolinium enhancement will reveal the presence of arachnoiditis. In olden days contrast myelography showed a characteristic picture of 'candle guttering' due to multiple levels of blocks and fragmentation of the dye column.

Treatment is largely medical, with antitubercular therapy and steroids being administered in the tubercular variety of the disease, and steroids and penicillin in the syphilitic variety. Hyalurinidase in the dose of 1500 units is injected intrathecally fortnightly, and if improvement is noted, the treatment should be continued till no further improvement occurs.

Tuberculoma usually shows central zone of caseating necrosis with capsule of collagenous tissue, epitheloid cells, multinucleated giant cells and mononuclear inflammatory cells with parenchymal oedema and astrocytic proliferation. Few bacilli may be found in the central necrotic area. They usually are found in cerebrum, cerebellum, subarachnoid spaces, subdural space, and epidural space. They are usually infratentorial in children. They usually coexist in 10 % of patients with tubercular meningitis. In HIV infected patients with tubercular meningitis, tuberculoma usually are not found. Tuberculin test in patients with tuberculoma is positive in 85 % of adults and 50 % of children, however, when HIV infection is present the tuberculin test is positive in only 20 % of cases. The chest radiograph shows tuberculosis in 30 to 80 % of patients. It presents as usually space occupying lesion with headaches, signs of increased intracranial tension such as papilloedema, seizures and focal neurological signs. CSF shows non-specific increase in proteins. Neuroimaging shows lesions either at cortico-medullary junctions or periventricular regions. On CAT scan they are usually solid enhancing lesions, ring enhancing lesions or mixed. There may be a central calcification surrounded by hypodense area with peripheral ring enhancement. Multiple conglomerate lesions like a bunch of grapes may be seen. On MRI in T1 isointense to grey matter with slightly hyperintense rim may be observed and on T2 non-caseating lesions are bright with nodular enhancement while caseating lesions vary from isointense to hypointense with rim enhancement and perilesional oedema. The differential diagnosis is sarcoidosis, cysticercosis or toxoplasmosis. Sometimes instead of tuberculoma a tubercular abscess may be found.

FUNGAL INFECTIONS OF CNS

The fungus is a nucleus bounded by an organised membrane with mitochondria. It divides by mitosis and has chitin as the major cell wall component. Chitinous wall and lack of mobility help to differentiate fungi from protozoa and absent chlorophyl help to differentiate from plants and algae. They are dimoprphic and capable of existing in yeast or filamentous forms. The yeast is a unicellular round or elongated structure and is able to reproduce itself by budding or fission. Filamentous forms grow by extension of tips to form tubular filamentous structures called hyphae. Hyphae develop septa that divide them into apparent segments. Parts of hyphae can form reproductive elements called spores, which are dispersed in the air by winds. Spores develop into yeast when infecting humans but remain filamentous in the laboratory. When spores enter lungs by inhalation, the localised lesion may remain asyptomatic. On occasion they reach the blood stream and overcome the reticuloendothelial, cellular or humoral defence system and penetrate the blood brain barrier or blood CSF barrier to reach the meninges or the parenchyma. In the CNS fungi cause meningitis, meningoencephalitis, granuloma and micro-abscess. The yeast phase causes meningitis and meningoencephalitis, while the filamentous forms are found in abscesses. The meningoencephalitis occurs when the fungus from the meninges invade the parenchyma through the Virchow-Robin spaces. Mucormycosis and aspergillus invade the blood vessels causing endarteritis and haemorrhage due to the rupture of the affected blood vessel. The meninges are infected by a variety of fungi, such as Cryptococcus neoformans, Coccidiodes immitis, Histoplasma capsulatum, Candida albicans, Sporothrix schenckii and Blastomyces dermatitis. Cryptococcus and Coccidiodes usually cause the meningoencephalitis while abscess formation and granulomas are seen with Zygomycetes (mucormycosis), Aspergillus Coccidiodes and Blastomyces. The fungal infection can occur at any age. In infants infection with Candida and Histoplasma capsulatum is common. While Candida infection is usually seen in young or old persons. Candida is also seen in malnourished people, diabetics, and when shunts and arterial or venous lines are inserted. During pregnancy Coccidiodes infection is usual. Cryptococcal infection occurs in young and middle aged. Sinuses, orbits and mastoids are commonly infected with Zygomycetis (Mucormycosis), Aspergillus and Blastomyces dermatitis. In immunodeficiency, Hodgkin's disease and patients with AIDS, infection with Cryptococcus, Histoplasma and Coccidiodes, Aspergillus and blastomycetes is generally encountered. Fungal meningitis and granulomas are common in patients affected with AIDS. Patients receiving cytotoxic chemotherapy and/or high doses of steroids are generally infected with Aspergillus, Candida or Zygomycetes species. Finally, in recipients of organ transplants, infection with Aspergillus, Candida, Cryptococcus, Coccidiodes, Histoplasma and Mucormycosis commonly occurs. Males are more affected than females.

Fungal infection usually occurs with indwelling catheters or shunts, in patients who are immunosuppressed for control of autoimmune diseases and transplant rejection or in patients receiving chemotherapy. It also occurs in patients with phagocyte function disorders and in patients with impairment of cell mediated immunity and finally in patients with granulocyte function disorders. Fungus may spread to CNS from, lungs, skin, sinuses and orbits, bone and joints, kidneys, liver and spleen. Chest radiogram, sputum culture, bronchoscopic aspiration and finally biopsy will help detect the pulmonary fungus infection. Joint radiographs and bone scan will reveal lesions in those sites.

Cryptococcal meningitis is usually subacute. Fever, headaches, nuchal pain, cranial nerve palsies and seizures are the common presenting symptoms. Further, anaemia, and raised WBC counts and erythrocyte sedimentation rate (ESR), are found with infection. The CSF is clear, colourless with increased WBC count of 20-1000 lymphocytes. Neutrophils are present in infections with Aspergillus, Mucormycosis and Blastomycosis. Eosinophils are seen in

Coccidiodes infection. The glucose content is minimally low and the proteins are raised to 50-1000 mg/dl. Gram stain is negative. India ink preparation will show Cryptococci. Fungal culture of CSF is positive in 40-50 % of cases. Fungal antigens, antibodies to fungi, complement fixation (CF); Elisa and immunodiffusion essay is used for the diagnosis. Immunodiffusion is used for diagnosis of Aspergillus, Candida, and Coccidiodes, CF, Elisa and immunodiffusion; all three can help in the diagnosis of Blastomycosis. CSF antigen is positive in Cryptococcal infection while CF and immunodiffusion is used for Histoplasma and only Elisa for S.Schenckii. At times meningeal biopsy may have to be resorted to for the diagnosis.

Amphotericin B is the treatment of choice. The peak serum levels occur after 6-8 hours. The drug is excreted in urine. There is blood brain barrier block and hence at times it may have to be introduced in the CSF via Ommaya reservoir. There is considerable toxicity following administration of intravenous Amphotericin. Idiosyncratic reaction or anaphylaxis may occur. Acute hepatic failure, seizures, ventricular fibrillation and cardiac arrest may follow. Fever, chills, rigors, nausea, vomiting and phlebitis may occur. Prolonged administration leads to anaemia, hypokalemia and nephrotoxicity. Lipid formulations of Amhotericin are better tolerated but they are very expensive. Flucytosine is given in combination for Cryptococcal, Candida and Aspergillus infection. It is absorbed rapidly from GI tract and excreted in urine. The half-life of the drug is 3-5 hours and hence, it is given in multiple doses. It crosses the blood brain barrier and 5 % CSF concentration is achieved. Rash, diarrhoea, hepatic dysfunction may occur as toxic reaction. When administered with Amphotericin, marrow suppression and thrombocytopenia have to be guarded against. Fluconazole is also useful for treatment of Cryptococcal meningitis and is ideal for prophylactic treatment to prevent recurrence. An intravenous and oral form of Itriconazole in cyclodextrins is useful in variety of fungal infection.

NEUROSYPHILIS

As the incidence of neurosyphilis has declined dramatically since the advent of penicillin, a medical student often does not get the opportunity to study a patient with this disease whilst on the clinical service.

The primary chancre is generally the first manifestation of acquired syphilis, treponema being already disseminated in various tissues of the body, with central nervous system involvement occurring in the second stage of the disease. The involvement is asymptomatic, but meningovascular syphilis may present at this stage. Meningovascular syphilis can be divided into two forms: the cranial and the spinal form. The cranial form includes syphilitic meningitis, and a 'stroke' like syndrome giving rise to hemiplegia. The spinal form consists of meningomyelitis, cervical pachymeningitis, syphilitic amyotrophy and radiculitis. Symptoms may develop a few months to a few years after the primary infection.

Acute syphilitic meningitis behaves like any other acute meningitis. The CSF shows polymorphonuclear pleocytosis, the proteins are increased, the glucose is usually normal and the VDRL reaction is strongly positive. The chronic variety presents with involvement of a single or multiple cranial nerves, with third fourth, sixth and eighth being commonly affected. Adhesions at the base lead to hydrocephalus and signs of increased intracranial pressure. If the meningitis is restricted to the convexity of the brain, headaches and focal seizures occur.

The typical vascular lesion of syphilis is an endarteritis, with the middle cerebral artery commonly affected, producing a contralateral hemiplegia and/or aphasia etc. The gumma is rare, produces signs of increased intracranial pressure with focal neurological deficit and the VDRL reaction is positive in the CSF. Adhesive arachnoiditis, gumma formation and endarteritis of the vasa nervorum can lead to lesions of the optic nerve and chiasma.

The course of meningomyelitis is subacute, with backache and root pains in the dorsal region. A spastic paraplegia develops with sphincter involvement and a thoracic sensory level. Involvement of anterior spinal artery spares the posterior columns while involvement of both anterior and posterior arteries lead to transverse myelitis. Erb's syphilitic paraplegia occurs 5 to 10 years after the primary infection. The symptoms are those of a gradually progressive spastic paraplegia with bladder involvement and impotency. VDRL reaction in the CSF is positive.

GENERAL PARALYSIS OF THE INSANE (GPI) and tabes dorsalis are not seen these days. GPI occurs 5 to 25 years after primary infection, frequently in males. The patient presents with ill-defined symptoms such as headaches, restlessness, insomnia, and loss of drive and changes in personality and mood. With progress of the disease the memory deteriorates with loss of judgement and lack of social behaviour such as grandiose delusions with blunting of affect. Seizures and focal neurological deficits then develop and patient may need to be institutionalised. The pupils show the classical Argyll Robertson abnormality, namely, small irregular pupils that do not react to light but react promptly to accommodation. The CSF shows mild to moderate increase of lymphocytes, proteins and gammaglobulins.

TABES DORSALIS is another parenchymal disease that occurs 10 to 15 years after the primary infection. It occurs around fifth decade with male predominance. The lesion is in the dorsal nerve roots and degeneration of the posterior column. Fibres subserving pain are the first to be involved, leading to characteristic lightening pains, which usually involve the sciatic nerve or the thoracic roots leading to girdle pains or the viscera giving visceral pain. With progress of the disease there is loss of deep sensation and squeezing the patient's calf or testes, no pain is felt. Loss of proprioception leads to positive Romberg's sign and ataxia worst at night and a high steppage gait. The tendon reflexes are absent. Marked hypotonia causes excessive joint movements causes destruction of the joints – the classical Charcot's joint.

TREATMENT of neurosyphilis consists of administration of intravenous penicillin G, 3 – 4 million units every 4 hours for 10 to 14 days or intramuscularly 2.4 million units of procaine penicillin G, four times a day for 14 days with oral 500 mg of Probenecid four times a day. Benzathine penicillin in the dose of 2.4 million units is given once a week for 3 to 4 weeks following procaine penicillin.

ENCEPHALITIS

The term encephalitis generally means a non-suppurative

inflammation of the brain caused by variety of agents such as viruses and fungi. Many viruses affect the nervous system, the common ones being Rabies in India (Rhabdo virus), the virus of Japanese B encephalitis (Arbo virus), the Polio, the Coxsackie and the Echo virus (Entero virus) and the viruses of measles (Myxo), Chicken-pox, Herpes simplex and Herpes zoster (Variola virus). To this list should now be added the Human Immuno-deficiency Virus I and II (HIV I & II). Infection by the Cytomegalo and Epstein-Barr viruses may simultaneously accompany the HIV infection. Of these Rabies, Japanese B and Entero viruses infect the nervous system directly, whilst CNS involvement in mumps, measles, variola-varicella group and HIV is secondary to a generalised infection.

NEUROLOGICAL ABNORMALITIES IN HIV INFECTION (AIDS):

It is said that approximately 60 million persons are living with HIV infection. As the name suggests the target of the virus in the human body is the immune system including lymphocytes, microglia and macrophages. Initially, in the early 80s the majority of humans infected with HIV were homosexual or bisexual males and patients with haemophilia and coronary artery by-pass surgery, who had received multiple transfusions. However, recently the incidence has increased in intravenous drug users and heterosexual females, their paramours and children born to them. In India, heterosexual transmission may be more common.

Primary HIV infection is also known as seroconversion stage which after a long period of time – over 10 years, terminates in AIDS and if not treated leads to death. The Centres for Disease Control (CDC), USA, developed the most widely used classification for HIV. The infection is divided into four groups:

Group I	Primary HIV infection
Group II	Asymptomatic phase
Group III	Persistent generalised lymphadenopathy
Group IV	Symptomatic infection
A	HIV wasting syndrome (AIDS) and constitutional disease
B	HIV encephalopathy (AIDS) and neurological disease
C1	Major opportunistic infections
C2	Minor opportunistic infections

D Cancers specified as AIDS defining
E Other conditions

The primary HIV infection represents acquisition of the virus and development of antibodies. The symptoms are like mild glandular fever or encephalopathy. Without a high index of suspicion, the diagnosis may be missed. Tests for antibodies and antigen should be carried out on serial blood samples. If these are negative, but the suspicion is high, HIV RNA polymerase chain reaction (PCR) is indicated. There may be high viral load and depression of CD4 count. Treatment with antiretroviral agents may prevent or delay the development of AIDS.

The asymptomatic stage can last for 10 years. The intention to treat will depend on CD4 count and viral load. The potential gain of therapy must be weighed against potential risks.

Persistent generalised lymphadenopathy may be a presenting feature of HIV infection in a person. The presence of this does not worsen the prognosis. Treatment again should be decided on CD4 count and viral load.

Apart from the immune system, the nervous system is the most commonly affected. The virus is neurotropic and invades the entire neuraxis early. The virus can be recovered from both central and peripheral nervous system. The CSF abnormalities occur in the early course of the infection and anti HIV antibodies develop. The central and peripheral nervous system dysfunction develops in the later stages of the disease, which may be due to chronic immunosuppression, or direct neurotropism of the virus and/or complications of the medical management. Though pathological lesions of the nervous system at autopsy are found in almost all patients with HIV infection, the symptoms of CNS and PNS involvement during life develop in 50 per cent of infected patients only.

With seroconversion, (HIV positive status), fever, headache, sore throat, myalgia, fatigue, anorexia, diarrhoea and skin rash may appear. The constitutional symptoms of fever and diarrhoea lasting for over a month with weight loss of over 10 % of base line, should make one suspect AIDS. As stated earlier at this stage many patients may have meningitis and this is the time when patients may have severe headaches. HIV antibodies and P24 antigen may be detected in the CSF at this stage. If there is high viral load, low CD4 count (less than 400), fungal or tubercle meningitis may be found. Even other viruses or parasites with low pathogenicity and virulence may invade at this stage. CAT scan and MRI examination may be carried out to exclude intracranial lesions. Due to drug abuse and alcoholism and malnutrition, one can encounter cerebral atrophy, but this atrophy is not the sign of 'AIDS dementia'. Patient's knowledge of sero-positivity may produce symptoms like dementia – such as memory loss, forgetfulness or impaired concentration but if friends and relatives have observed no abnormality and the cognitive tests are normal, the pressure of depression is inferred. This needs to be identified and attended.

The early neurological manifestation may be related to cranial nerves – bilateral facial weakness with Guillaine-Barre (acute inflammatory demyelinating polyneuropathy) like symptoms or mononeuritis multiplex or brachial neuritis. Serological tests for other infections like herpes simplex virus or cytomegalo-virus should be conducted and excluded following which treatment with plasmapharesis or intravenous immunoglobulin should be given. Corticosteroids should be avoided.

Seizures – generalised or focal may develop during the course of HIV infection. Focal seizures are usually due to Toxoplasma, tuberculoma or lymphoma. Focal neurological signs will be present on neurological examination and the imaging studies will reveal the presence of one of the above lesions. The generalised seizures may be due to metabolic changes, alcohol effect or complication of anti HIV virus therapy. Generalised seizures may be due to the infection. Anticonvulsants are indicated to control the seizures. However, Carbamazepine and Valproic acid should be avoided as they have toxic effects on the bone marrow. Phenytoin has interaction with protease inhibitors. Apart from the newer antiepileptics like Gabapentin, Lamotrigine and Topiramate, in our country, Phenobarbitone with its low cost, is also an option.

With development of immunosuppression, decline of cognitive function such as reading, concentration, losing track of conversation and slowness of thinking, may be observed. Motor symptoms like stiffness of legs, change in handwriting may be present. This association has poor prognosis. Chorea, dystonia and tremors may also be associated. However, these dyskinesias can be drug induced. Treatment these days has reduced the incidence of HIV dementia. The CAT findings are of enlarged ventricular and subarachnoid spaces with multiple hypodense, non-contrast enhanced, white matter, basal ganglia and thalamic abnormalities. On MRI high signal intensity without contrast is noted in the same areas.

Pathologically multiple nodules consisting of gliosis and microglia, macrophages and multinucleated giant cells are encountered. The white matter pallor is not due to demyelination but more likely due to cytokine related inflammation and viral penetration.

Myopathy, myelitis due to HIV and other opportunistic viruses and ischaemic or haemorrhagic strokes are also encountered in AIDS.

Opportunistic infection due to viruses, fungi, parasites and bacteria is common. They either cause meningitis or space occupying lesions. Cryptococcus is diagnosed by positive India ink preparation in CSF and elevated antigen in CSF and blood. Fluconazole and Amphotericin B with or without Flucytosine is used to treat Cryptococcal meningitis. There is 20 % mortality. Oral Candida may be asymptomatic. In severe infection, local Nystatin is used, with oral Ketoconazole or Fluconazole. This will take care of oropharyngeal or oesophageal candidiasis. Long-term maintenance therapy may become necessary to prevent recurrences. Candidal vulvovaginitis and be recurrent and is treated with topical applications of Clotrimazole or Miconazole. Pneumocystis carinii pneumonia is very common in developed countries, while in India tuberculosis is commonly encountered. Hence, prophylaxis with Co-trimoxazole is essential for Pneumocystis infection. The infection is treated by Co-trimoxazole (15-20 mg/kg/day), or Clindamycin 600 mg 6 hourly or Trimethoprim (20mg/kg/day) with Dapsone 100 mg daily have been advocated. Toxoplasmosis is the common cause of ring enhancing lesion on contrast CT. The treatment with Sulphadiazine (4-6 G/day), Pyrimethamine (50-100 mg/day) and Folinic acid (15 mg/day) should be started early. Prophylaxis and maintenance treatment for prolonged period is imperative. Raw or undercooked meat and vegetables should be avoided to prevent infection.

Cryptosporidiosis infection usually causes self-limiting gastrointestinal illness. Symptomatic treatment with antidiarrhoeal and antiemetic agents with fluid, electrolyte and nutritional support should be provided. In severe infection, Spiramycin or Erythromycin may be needed.

Herpes simplex and Cytomegalovirus are the common opportunistic viruses. Cutaneous herpes is treated by Acyclovir 200 mg, five times a day orally for 5 to 7 days. It can also be given intravenously if there is encephalitis, in the dose of 10-15 mg/kg every 8 hours for 5-7 days. Cytomegalovirus infection needs more aggressive treatment with Ganciclovir in the dose of 5 mg/kg intravenously, twice a day for 14 to 21 days. Cidofovir and Foscarnet both nephrotoxic drugs may be needed if Ganciclovir does not work. Cidofovir is administered in the dose of 5mg/kg once a week for two weeks, with Probenecid and hydration to prevent nephrotoxicity. Foscarnet is used in the dose of 180 mg/kg/day for 14-21 days. The dose being adjusted according to the renal symptoms. The maintenance therapy is continued with Ganciclovir 3 mg daily orally.

Tuberculosis is the common bacterial infection and is treated with Rifampicin, Isoniazide, Pyrazinamide and Ethambutol. Rifampicin has drug interaction with protease inhibitors and non-nucleoside reverse transcriptase inhibitors. Disseminated lesions with Mycobacterium avium cause considerable morbidity and mortality. Primary prophylaxis with Rifabutin (300 mg daily) or Clarithromycin (500 mg twice daily) or Azithromycin (200 mg once weekly), should be considered to prevent this high mortality and morbidity. Salmonella and Campylobacter infections are treated with Ciprofloxacin. Recently, an interesting observation has been made. Patients having hepatitis G infection, which hardly causes any disease or hepatic damage, has decreased susceptibility to HIV virus and patients with hepatitis G infection, suffering from AIDS live longer. It is thought that the hepatitis G virus directly prevents the replication of HIV virus on the other hand HSV2 infection increases the risk of HIV transmission 2 to 4 times. Hence, it is advisable to give chronic

Acyclovir therapy to HSV2 virus carriers.

The treatment for HIV is usually started when the CD4 count falls below 350. The HIV infection is treated with combination of reverse transcriptase inhibitors and the protease inhibitors

Table 5.1.

Reverse Transcriptase Inhibitors

Name	Indications	Dose	Toxicity
Zidovudine (AZT)	For HIV	200 mg three times 300 mg twice	Granulopenia Anaemia, Myopathy, Lactic acidosis, headache, hepatomegaly
	Prevention of Maternal-foetal transmission	100mgx 5/day till initial labour then 2mg/kg over 1 hour iv followed by 1mg/kg iv until clamping of cord. Infant 2mg/kg 6 hourly orally within 12 hours or 1.5mg/kg 6hrly iv over 30 minutes.	
Didanosine videx (ddl)	Combination AZT+ ddl	>60kg 200mg bd <60kg 125mg bd	Pancreatitis,neuropathy, LFT deranged
Zalcitabine (ddc)	Combination Inferior to AZT	>60kg 40mg bd <60kg 30mg bd	Pancreatitis, neuropathy
Stavudine	who has recd. previous AZT	>60kg 40mg bd <60kg 30mg bd	same as above
Lamivudine 3TC	Combination Superior to AZT	150 mg bd	
Abacavir	Combination Abacavir+AZT+3TC Indinavir+AZT+3TC	300 mg bd	Hypersensitivity reaction, fever, rash, nausea, vomiting, fatigue, loss of appetite
Delavirdin Rescriptor	Combination With AZT	400mg tid	Skin rash, abnormal LFT
Efavirenz	Combination efavirenz+AZT+3TC Indinavir+AZT+3TC	600mg qid	Rash, dysphoria Abnormal LFT
<u>Protease inhibitor</u> Saquinar Mesylate Inviran hard gel capsule	Combination	600mg 8hrly	Diarrhoea, nausea headache, hyperglycemia, lipid abn.
Fortovase Soft gel capsule	Combination	1200mg bd	Same as above

Ritonavir Norvir	Combination with nucleoside analogues	600mg bd	Same as above interaction with Saquinavir
Indinavir		800mg 8hrly	Nephrolithiasis Hyperglycemia Hyperbilirubinemia Lipid abnormality
Nelfinavir Mesylate Viracept		750mg tds 1250mg bd	Diarrheoa, hyper-glycemia, lipid abnormalities
Amprenavir	+AZT+3TC Superior to AZT+3TC	1200mg bd	Nausea, vomiting rash. oral paraesthesia, LFT increased, hyperglycemia lipid abnormalities
Lopinavir Ritonavir	+d4T+3TC Superior to Nelfinavir +d4T+3TC	100-400mg bd	diarrhoea, hyper glycemia, lipid abn normalities

Following few points in CSF examination help in differentiating bacterial, viral, fungal and tubercular meningitis.

Table 5.2

CSF In Various Meningitis

CSF parameters	Bacterial	Viral	Fungal	TBM
Opening pressure	>180	Normal	Variable	>180
WBC count cells/mm²	1,000- 10,000	<300	50 -4000	50 - 500
Neutrophils	>80 %	<20 %	usually less<50%	<20%
Protein mg	100 – 500	often normal	Elevated	150 –200
Glucose	<40	>40	usually <40	<40

Antigen +ve and antibody titres in fungus 75% in cryptococcus, 50% in Histoplasma, 45% in coccidiodes, 40% in candida, less often in other fungi.

Prions +ve in 90 % sporadic and 10 % in inherited.

CSF fluorescent treponemal antibody-absorption test (FTA-ABS) & CSF micro haem agglutination test for treponema pallidum.

PCR for viral Herpes simplex encephalitis +ve in 10-20 %, VZV, Epstein Barr, Polyoma virus causing progressive multifocal leucoencephalopathy called J.C. virus 70 –90 %.CMV 80 –100 % sensitivity & 75 % specificity.

JAPANESE B ENCEPHALITIS: This occurs in epidemic but is also endemic in northern, eastern and central regions of the country. It is due to a Flavi virus. Another Arbo virus that is common to south India is the Kyasanur forest disease virus. Birds, especially pigeons are the primary host of Japanese B encephalitis, whilst monkeys are the host for Kyasanur forest virus. Mosquitoes are the vectors for Japanese B virus whilst fleas, ticks and mosquitoes are the vectors for Kyasanur forest virus. The Japanese B encephalitis is usually seen in children. In the initial stage of viraemia the patient complaints of fever, body ache, lethargy and generalised weakness. Headaches, vomiting, restlessness, irritability, delirium and drowsiness herald the onset of encephalitis. Frequent seizures occur and coma ensues. Behavioural disturbances and thought disorders may occur in the early stages of the illness, leading to an erroneous diagnosis of a psychiatric disease. Tremors, parkinsonian features and cranial nerve palsies are reported. Focal neurological signs in the form of hemiplegia or monoplegia may be present. Signs of meningeal involvement are minimal or absent. In the final stage of the disease signs of decortication and decerebration appear. The mortality rate is high.

CSF examination shows a mild lymphocytic pleocytosis with minimal elevation of the proteins. The glucose is normal. Antibodies to the virus are detected. The EEG shows generalised slowing with focal or generalised epileptiform discharges. The CAT scan may show hypodensity in the white matter with enhancement of the gyri on contrast. The diagnosis is simple when the epidemic is raging. Sporadic case needs detailed study with history of exposure, lack of meningeal signs and typical CSF with raised antibody titre for Japanese B virus, EEG and imaging findings. Toxic encephalopathies can be differentiated by history of exposure to toxins, and metabolic encephalopathies are associated with features of primary involvement of liver, kidneys etc. It is preventable by vaccination.

Treatment is largely symptomatic with steroids providing dubious benefit. Hyperthermia, restlessness, irritability and seizures should be treated with appropriate measures. The morbidity of encephalitis is high, with chorea, extrapyramidal problems like parkinsonism, sleep disturbances, epilepsy, intellectual deficits and hemiplegia being prominent sequelae.

Post-infectious encephalitis shows similar clinical features and occurs either during the course of the infectious fever or rarely immediately after the infection. Rarer still, there is only history of contact with a case of infectious fever. Encephalitis, encephalomyelitis and peripheral neuropathies may occur with measles, mumps, variola, varicella and Epstein-Barr infection. PCR helps in the diagnosis of Epstein-Barr infection and Acyclovir or Ganciclovir are useful for treatment. Varicella Zoster virus produces vasculitis due to which haemorrhagic lesions, or mixed ischaemic and demyelinating lesions occur. Periventriculitis and ventriculitis also occur. The symptoms are headaches, malaise, confusion, delirium and seizures. The CNS affection can occur after days or months after the eruptions disappear, though the average is 9-10 days. The treatment consists of Valaciclovir, Famciclovir or Ganciclovir.

Cytomegalovirus infection is acquired through oral or respiratory secretions and through contact with infected urine or faeces, blood, semen and breast milk. A large population has already been exposed by the age of 50 years. The virus causes parenchymal cellular necrosis, leading to formation of microglial nodules and also produces ventriculoencephalitis. The encephalitis and ventriculoencephalitis produces confusion, disorientation, apathy, psychomotor slowing and few days to week later cranial nerve palsies.

HERPES SIMPLEX ENCEPHALITIS is the commonest non-epidemic form of encephalitis. It can occur at any age but is more frequently seen in children. The virus has predilection for temporal lobe, behavioural disturbances and seizures are common, as are focal neurological signs. There is massive swelling of the temporal lobes, and consequent rise in intracranial pressure. Isolation of virus by immunofluorescent techniques or PCR, detection of antibodies in serum and CSF are diagnostic tools. Prompt administration of Acyclovir in the dosage mentioned earlier reduces mortality and morbidity.

POLIOMYELITIS: Availability of vaccine and massive programme to eliminate poliomyelitis has eventually paid dividends.

The oral polio vaccine is given at 6 months of age and repeated after 6 weeks and 6 months. A booster dose is given when the child enters the school and at 15 to 20 years of age. Today, the students will hardly get a chance to see a case of polio. Pathologically the lesions involve mainly the anterior horn cells of the spinal cord and the cells of bulbar motor cranial nerve nuclei. Poliovirus is an enterovirus and enters the human body through the gatrointestinal tract. The prodormal illness consists of fever, malaise, coryza and gastrointestinal disturbances for 2 to 3 days. The symptoms abate for a few days, before the start of preparalytic stage. The temperature rises; the patient has a severe headache and stiffness of the neck. There may be severe pain in the limbs, and even a minimal movement of the limb causes excruciating pain; hence the patient resists any attempts at movement of the limb. Then the paralytic stage sets in, the fever drops and the pain abates. Motor paralysis which is asymmetric and may be localised or wide spread ensues. The affected muscles are flaccid, weak, and atrophic. Tendon reflexes are lost in the affected muscles. There is no sensory loss and fasciculation are rare. In some patients, the paralysis may spread to involve bulbar muscles, causing respiratory distress and difficulty with articulation or swallowing. Patient may need assisted ventilation and a tracheostomy. Patients with bulbar paralysis have high mortality and morbidity. CSF shows a polymorphonuclear pleocytosis in the first week changing to lymphocytic preponderance, with elevated proteins and normal glucose levels. The virus can be isolated from the stool, serum and CSF. Viral antibody titre rises.

Acute infectious polyneuritis is differentiated by the symmetric distribution of weakness. In 1971 and 1981 epidemics of acute **HAEMORRHAGIC CONJUNCTIVITIS** have occurred in India. Extensive polio like paralysis has been reported as sequelae. Males were more commonly affected and there was no age preference. In some cases, cranial nerves, especially the seventh nerve was involved.

Intramuscular injections are strictly avoided. The pain is relieved by immobilisation of limbs and analgesics. Management consists of prevention of contractures, with intense rehabilitation measures.

With the evolution of the concept of slow virus infection from the study of the disease called 'Kuru' in New Guinea, more slow virus diseases in humans have come to light. **SUBACUTE SCLEROSING PANENCEPHALITIS (SSPE)** is commoner as compared to **SUBACUTE SPONGIFORM ENCEPHALOPATHY (SSE)**, which is extremely rare. SSE can be sporadic, acquired (iatrogenic) or familial. The familial form is inherited as autosomal dominant, due to mutation of the gene that encodes the Prion protein. Recently, bovine spongiform encephalopathy has been recognised, which can infect humans. Initially the SSE was seen in goat and sheep known as Scrapie. The other diseases are Gerstmann-Straussler-Scheinker disease and Fatal familial insomnia, which are due to mutation of Prion protein gene.

Prion protein is defined as 27-30 kDa protein resistant to limited proteolysis. Protease sensitive form or Prion protein is a highly conserved protein present in normal individuals, in many tissues and abundant in neurones. Prion protein resistant to proteases is present in diseased brains because it takes one of several configuration that is different from the normal. The abnormal form resists denaturation, fixation, digestion and charastically aggregates. It enters the CNS and serves as a catalyst that changes the normal Prion protein to the abnormal variety. The gene for prion protein is on the short arm of chromosome 20. Infectious prions travel to germinal centres of the lymph nodes from where it infects the CNS via B -lymphocytes.

The incidence of SSPE is on the decline due to use of measles virus vaccine, but cases are still seen. The disease occurs around 6-14 years of age. There is history of measles infection in childhood. It begins with gradual progression of intellectual deterioration. Few months later the patient develops myoclonic jerks, which are multifocal. Seizures occur. From then on the course is progressively downhill, with marked mental deterioration, aphasia, apraxia and quadriplegia, leading to a vegetative state and death, within few months to few years of the onset of the disease. The EEG shows characteristic recurring periodic discharges. As yet there is no known treatment of the disease.

JAKOB-CRUETZFELDT DISEASE: It is seen in 1 per million population affects the central nervous system and has a subacute progressive course. It can be either sporadic which is around 90% of all cases, acquired is only 5% and genetic is around 15%. Infection is transmissible to animals and in humans after surgery and implantation of dural grafts or following growth hormone administration. The sporadic or genetic disease presents with progressive dementia or ataxia or a mixed picture. Parkinsonian features and myoclonus are also prominent clinical features. On examination, evidence of pyramidal as well as extrapyramidal systems involvement is obtained. Signs of lower motor neurone involvement are seen in the later stages of the disease. Once again the EEG shows the characteristic periodic discharges in the frontal regions recurring every ½ to 2 seconds, with generalised slowing which is seen in both sporadic and acquired disease. MRI shows hyperintensities in the caudate, putamen, globus pallidus and thalamus in T2 sequences. The CSF shows 14-3-3 protein. Prion protein gene (PRNP) has been identified on short arm of chromosome 20 and can help in the molecular diagnosis. The acquired disease usually presents with ataxia and minimal dementia and personality changes. The patient usually dies within six months of the onset of the disease. Recently, newer form of Jakob-Creutzfeldt disease has been described. It is transmitted by the bovine spongiform encephalopathy prions. It is noted that it occurs more commonly in humans who lack the HLA complex DQ7. It occurs in younger generation and presents with prominent psychiatric symptoms. It is not reported from India.

CYSTICERCOSIS is seen through out the country but in southern and northern states of India, it is maximal. The causative agent is Cysticercus cellulosae – a larval form of tapeworm – Taenia solium. The infection develops by eating inadequately cooked infected pork or contaminated food and vegetables due to unhygienic habits. It may present in variety of ways. Patients usually present with seizures, focal or generalised, or with evidence of encephalitis, meningo-encephalitis or signs of increased intracranial tension. Multiple small nodules may be detected elsewhere in the body or radiological examination of the extremities may reveal calcified cysts. The imaging techniques have helped to pick up single ring enhancing lesions or multiple cysts. The former has to be differentiated from other granulomatous lesions. Usually the scolex is seen in the cystic lesion. The treatment consists of Albandazole in the dose of 15mg/kg/day for 30 days or Praziquintal in the dose of 50mg/kg/day for 15 days if the cysts are present in various stages of development. Treatment at times leads to meningeal inflammatory reaction, which may intensify the occlusive endarteritis. The single lesion may not be treated. Symptomatic treatment inclusive of anti epileptic drugs is imperative.

CEREBRAL MALARIA: Malaria, which was once almost eradicated from India, has again made its presence felt. Cerebral malaria occurs with infection by the Falciparum strain. The diagnosis of cerebral malaria is not easy, and is made on presumptive evidence. If a patient with malarial fever develops signs of confusion, restlessness, or coma and convulsions, this diagnosis should be considered. On examination will have generalised hypertonia with opisthotonus, and later decerebration and decortication. He may also have internuclear ophthalmoplegia, with dysconjugate gaze. However, the Doll's eye movements, the corneal, conjunctival and pupillary reflexes are preserved. He will have strenuous breathing.When blood smears are positive for plasmodium falciparum infection, a diagnosis of cerebral malaria should be considered and the patient treated. Prompt response to therapy would further substantiate the diagnosis. However, it is wiser to exclude other causes of coma or encephalopathy at the same time.

The treatment consists of intramuscular injection of 200 mg of chloroquine base (250 mg Of hydrochloride), half the dose is given in each buttock. This may be repeated every 6 hours and in the first 24 hours the dose of Chloroquine base should not exceed 800 mg. Intravenous infusion of glucose saline should be started. Dexamethasone is not recommended, as it tends to increase the mortality. However, to reduce intracranial pressure, Mannitol may be used. If the falciparum strain is resistant to Chloroquine, Quinine is given in the dose of 20mg/kg as IV infusion over 4 hours and watch kept on the pulse and blood pressure. It can also be given as intramuscular injection in the dose of diluted 20mg/kg. However, it is painful and may cause muscle necrosis. It is preferable to treat the patient in an intensive care unit. At times facilities for IV quinine may not be available or the falciparum infection is resistant to quinine, a new drug Artimisinine has been introduced which can be given intramuscular or orally. In India Arteether (called E MAL or Falcy) is available and is given in the dose of 150mg daily for 3 days orally. The intramuscular dose is 3.2mg/kg followed by 1.2 mg/kg every 24 hours for 4 days. Another compound of Artimisinine called Artimether (Larither) is also available. It can be given orally in the dose of 80 mg twice a day for the first day and then 80 mg once a day for 4 days or intramuscularly in the dose of 80mg twice a day for 3 days. For prevention of recurrence a combination of Pyrimethamine and Sulfadoxin (Reziz forte –750mg of Sulphadoxin and 25 mg of Pyrimethamine) is given in the dose of 2 tablets twice a day for one day.

CHAPTER VI EPILEPSIES

The word epilepsy is derived from the Greek words, 'epi' meaning upon and 'lepos' meaning to seize. In ancient times an attack of seizure was believed to be due to the patient's soul being seized by a demon or god or inflicted or possessed by a supernatural power. In India, the popular belief was that the angry ancestral spirit or soul entered the patient's body and attempts were made to drive out the same. On the other hand, in Europe, there were some who believed that epilepsy was a Holy sickness, or Divine Disease as Alexander the Great, Julius Caesar, Napoleon Bonaparte, Charles Dickens, Dostoyevsky and van Gogh suffered from it. It is said that Shri Ramkrishna Paramhans also suffered from epilepsy. It was Hippocrates and Shrushrusha in India discounted the myths and were the first to observe that seizures originated from the brain.

Hughlings Jackson laid the foundation for the modern understanding of epilepsy. He published a series of brilliant papers in the nineteenth century, and delineated the different types of seizures. The introduction of electroencephalography (EEG) helped to understand the basic electrophysiological mechanisms of epilepsy. The recent advances in experimental neurology, study of neurotransmitters, electron microscopy, MRI, positron emission tomography and other advances in technology has helped to a large extent to understand the basic mechanisms of epilepsy and thereby help evolve newer pharmaceutical agents to treat epilepsy.

According to World Health Organization 50 million people of all age groups around the world suffer from epilepsy. Up to 70 % of these can be made seizure free with treatment.

It is important that the student realises at the outset the difference between the terms 'seizure' and 'epilepsy'. A seizure is due to a sudden, excessive, rapid discharge of the neurones by variety of metabolic, traumatic or toxic causes. (Table 6.1)

Table 6.1

Common Drugs Associated With Seizures

Analeptics	Aminophylline, Ephidrine, Amphetamine
Analgesics	Pethidine, Cocaine, Dextroproproxyphane
Antibiotics	Benzylpeniciline, Ampicillin, Cycloserine, INH, Nalidexic acid
Antidepressants	Amitryptilline, Imipramine
Antipsychotics	Chlorpromazine, Lithium
Radiographic contrast media	Metrizamide
Miscellaneous	D-Penicillamine, Baclofen, Folate, Piperazine, Cyclosporin, Hyperbaric oxygen

Epilepsy on the other hand, is the occurrence of two or more seizures recurring over a period of time, that do not occur in relation to any given factors like drug withdrawal or an acute illness. A single seizure occurs in approximately 7 % of population at one time in their life.

FEBRILE SEIZURES are seizures that occur between the ages of 3 months and 5 years. The seizure is accompanied by a rise in temperature and it is not a symptom of recognised acute neurological illness. For it to be a febrile seizure, it should occur within 12 hours of the rise of temperature. The seizure may occur once or recur. A third of patients have one recurrence while 10% have three or more. There is generally a family history of febrile seizures and/or epilepsy. In simple febrile seizure, the seizure is generalised tonic-clonic in nature, is not prolonged and the child regains consciousness immediately after the seizure. On the other hand the complex febrile seizure is partial at onset, lasts for 15-30 minutes and the child may not regain consciousness immediately. Absence seizures are not associated with febrile seizures. Epilepsy occurs in 10-15 % of patients with simple or complex febrile seizures with a positive family history of either febrile seizures or epilepsy. Despite the above, it is now observed, that at the time of diagnosis of epilepsy in children, there is a notable lack of association between febrile seizures and partial seizures, or localisation related epilepsy or temporal lobe epilepsy. If any relationship is encountered, it is believed that this is due to pre existing pathology or susceptibility. Substantial part of the risk is inherent in the individual and not febrile seizures per se. Moreover, early treatment can prevent recurrent febrile seizures but this does not decrease the risk of occurrence of unprovoked seizures or epilepsy. The management of recurrent febrile seizures consists of reducing the fever as soon as it is noted by use of Paracetamol and/or cold sponges. Oral or rectal Diazepam (1mg/kg in three divided doses) can be administered with the rise in temperature, to prevent febrile seizures. Phenobarbitone orally, in the dose of 10-20 mg/kg in three divided doses may be tried and if found effective, it could be continued till 5years of age. If it produces restlessness or any other toxic symptoms, the other drug commonly used in infants and young children is Valproic acid.

The prevalence of epilepsy is said to be around 6 per thousand. The figure could be higher in poor and uneducated population. The recent figures from Kerala for prevalence are 4.9 per thousand, 6.5 per thousand in population of 10-19 years of age. The overall prevalence rate in India is 5.59/1000, in men around 6.05/1000 as compared to 5.18/1000 in women. The prevalence is higher in urban population (6.34/1000) compared to rural (4.94/1000). However, 74 percent constitute rural population where a facility for proper treatment of epilepsy is lacking. Of the total projected population in India in 2001, there will be 5.5 million epileptics. Half million new cases occur every year. The prevalence in India is a little higher than Western Hemisphere due to illiteracy and poverty, which leads to delay in treatment. Generalised epilepsy is around 60 % and localisation related around 30 %.

There are many epileptic syndromes, which are inherited. However, the role of inheritance in other types of epilepsy is still controversial. Eighty per cent of siblings of patients with absence attacks demonstrate typical spike and wave pattern in their EEG. As yet there are no suitable controlled studies that identify the risk of developing seizures or epilepsy and the final word on genetic counselling is awaited.

The causes of seizures are tabulated below:

Table 6.2

Causes Of Seizures

Infections	Meningitis – especially tuberculous in our country. Encephalitis, Brain abscess, Tuberculoma and parasitic infestations like Cysticercosis.
Vascular	Cerebral infarction, Subarachnoid haemorrhage, Hypertensive encephalopathy, Stokes-Adams syndrome, Systemic lupus erythematosus, Arterio-venous malformations.
Metabolic	Hypoglycaemia, Uraemia, Hypoxia, Alkalosis, Pyridoxine deficiency, Hypocalcaemia, Porphyria, Eclampsia, Phenylketonuria.
Trauma	Concussion, Contusion, Penetrating head injury, Subdural haematoma.
Toxins	Heavy metals -arsenic, lead, Organo-phosphorus and Organochlorine compounds used as insecticides, Carbon monoxide, Alcohol, Drugs: Anti-depressants, Isoniazide, Cardiazol, and Nikethamide.
Tumours	Primary and secondary
Congenital Anomalies	Cerebral diplegia, Tuberous sclerosis, Cerebral dysgenesis, Hydrocephalus
Degeneration	Friedreich's ataxia, Ramsay Hunt syndrome, Lipid storage disorders, Mitochondrial cytopathy, Schilder's disease, Picks and Alzheimer's disease.
Miscellaneous	Fever, Photo stimulation, Television, etc.

Seizures are classified according to the classification suggested by the International League against Epilepsy (ILAE). They are divided into two broad categories – Generalised and partial. Generalised seizures are those seizures in which the onset is bilateral and results in loss of consciousness. The main types of generalised seizures are:

1) Absence seizures
2) Tonic-clonic seizures
3) Myoclonic seizures
4) Atonic seizures

Partial seizures are those seizures in which the seizure begins locally either clinically or on the EEG. Partial seizures are further classified into *Simple* partial seizures where consciousness is not impaired during the seizure and *Complex* partial seizures where is impairment of consciousness during the seizure. In clinical practise it is difficult to determine the loss of consciousness or awareness during a partial seizure.

Consciousness is defined as loss of awareness or responsiveness or both of the patients to external stimuli. The degree may vary. Sometimes, during the seizure awareness may be present but responsiveness is lost.

In 1989, ILAE reclassified epilepsies and epilepsy syndromes as under:

Table 6.3

Classification of Epilepsies

I. Localisation related - (focal, local partial)

A. *Idiopathic* – age related
   1. Benign childhood epilepsy with centro-temporal spikes
   2. Childhood epilepsies with occipital paroxysm
   3. Benign psychomotor childhood epilepsy

B. *Symptomatic* – Syndrome of great individual variation

II. Generalised epilepsies and syndromes (Grand-mal Petit-mal)

A. *Idiopathic* – age related
   1. Benign neonatal familial convulsions
   2. Benign neonatal convulsions
   3. Benign myoclonic epilepsy in infancy
   4. Childhood absence epilepsy (Petit mal, pyknolepsy)
   5. Juvenile absences
   6. Generalised Tonic-clonic seizures
   7. Absences
   8. Myoclonus
      a. Cortical Reflex myoclonus
      b. Reticular Reflex myoclonus
      c. Primary generalised epileptic myoclonus

9. Epilepsy with Grand mal seizures on awakening
10. Tonic and Atonic seizures

B. *Symptomatic or both*
   1. West's syndrome (Infantile spasms)
   2. Lennox-Gastaut syndrome
   3. Epilepsy with myoclonic-astatic syndrome
   4. Epilepsy with myoclonic syndrome

C. *Symptomatic*
   1. Early myoclonic encephalopathy non-specific cause
   2. Specific syndromes - Epilepsy may complicate many disease states

III. Epilepsies and syndromes undetermined whether they are Focal or Generalised

A. *With both focal and generalised seizures*
   1. Neonatal seizures
   2. Severe myoclonic epilepsy in infancy
   3. Epilepsy with continuous spike-waves during slow wave sleep
   4. Acquired epileptic aphasia – Landau-Kleffner syndrome

B. *Without unequivocal generalised or focal features*

IV. Special syndromes

A. *Situation related syndromes*
   1. Febrile convulsions
   2. Seizures related to other identifiable features, stress, hormones, drugs, alcohol, sleep

B. *Isolated unprovoked epilepsies*

C. *Epilepsies characterised by specific modes of seizure precipitation*
   1. Photic stimulation, Hot water epilepsy, Sleep loss.

D. *Chronic progressive epilepsy – epileptia partialis continua*

ABSENCE SEIZURES (Petit-Mal): These seizures are common in childhood, with the age of onset being 5-7 years. They comprise between 3-10 % of all seizures, but are less common in India than in Western countries. The seizures begin and end suddenly. There is no aura, no massive spasms, no formed speech, and no post ictal phase. The average duration of an absence is 10 seconds, with spells longer than 45 seconds being very unusual. The simple absence with just impaired responsiveness occurs in less than 10% of absences. The frequency of absences varies between 25 to over 100 seizures a day. The most common spell involves mild clonic activity, and simple automatisms like lip licking, and lip smacking and/or pill rolling movement. Automatisms are involuntary motor acts that occur during a seizure and are followed by amnesia for the event. Patients may have generalised tonic-clonic seizure as well. In complex partial seizures, loss of awareness or responsiveness may be seen, during which usually patient has a staring look, smacking of the lips or a little dribble of saliva from the mouth. There may be an aura before the impairment of consciousness. Such attacks occur once or twice a day and may not recur for days.

Absence status is usually precipitated by drug exposure or drug withdrawal. It is sometimes inconspicuous to both patient and the physician. Manifestations during absence status range from behavioural change to prolonged confusional state with partial recollection of events. During absence status patient is unable to sustain attention, he lacks initiative and has defect in planning, perseverates, and he has paucity of speech and memory disturbance. During the status he is able to carry out automatic activity and is able to execute complex commands. He is able to retain information in form of complex sentences and even calculate. It is difficult to differentiate from complex non-convulsive status of frontal lobe origin.

In classical Petit Mal, the EEG shows typical 3 per second generalised spike and wave discharge (Fig 6.1). Thalamo-cortical circuits that participate in production of sleep spindles are involved. Synaptic synchronisation during the waking state may produce absence seizures. The electrical activity also begins and ends abruptly like the clinical attack. EEG changes always present during the attack. Hyperventilation almost always precipitates an attack of absence. It is interesting to note that tasks ordered during a spike and wave discharge can be carried out after the discharge is over. Secondly, patient is able to continue counting, during the period of electrical discharge. The prognosis for remission from these seizures depends upon the normalcy of mental development and neurological examination, the typicality of the EEG findings, the absence of generalised tonic-clonic seizures, and a negative family history of seizures. If all four factors are present, there is a 90 % chance of remission by the time patient has reached puberty.

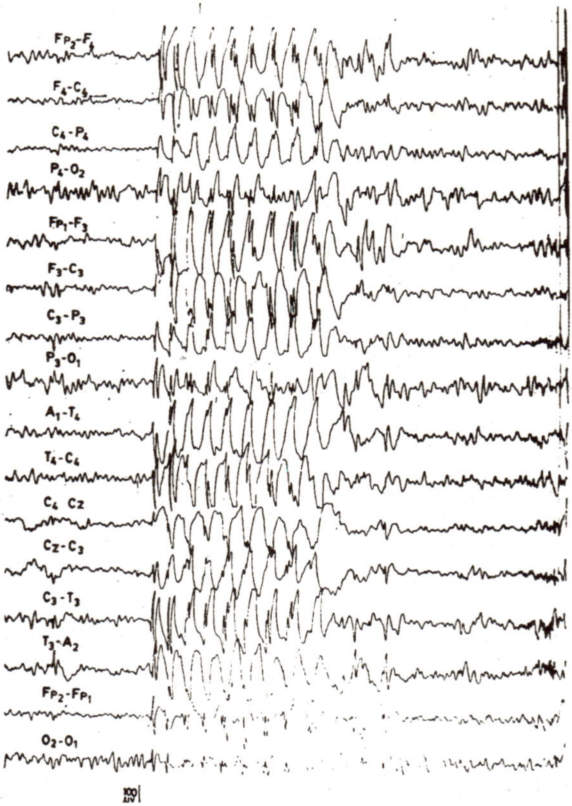

Fig 6.1 An EEG showing 3/ sec, spike and wave discharges

Absences are relatively easy to treat, with Valproate (20 –30 mg/ kg per day in divided doses) and Ethosuximide (now not available in India). Both are very effective in controlling the spells. Carbamazepine, a widely used first line anti epileptic and other newer antiepileptics either have no effect or some may even worsen the seizures. Lamotrigine may have beneficial effect.

GENERALISED TONIC-CLONIC SEIZURE (Grand-mal seizure)

This is the seizure that the layman describes as "convulsion". The seizure type can be seen at any age barring the first month of life (see later), and can be precipitated by stress, undue fatigue, and lack of sleep, fasting, and withdrawal from alcohol. Some patients report increase in seizure frequency in the pre-menstrual period (catamenial epilepsy).

The attack begins suddenly, the patient losing consciousness, and falling to the ground. An 'epileptic cry' is produced in most patients as the air is expressed out of the glottis due to tonic spasms of the respiratory muscles.

There is tonic extension of the limbs, followed by a phase of clonic contraction. In the tonic phase the limbs are extended and rigid with opisthotonus whilst in clonic phase there is alternate contraction and relaxation of the muscles. The eyeballs roll up, the tongue is protruded and hence may be bitten, there is frothing at mouth, and the patient may be incontinent of urine and faeces. The patient is amnestic for the attack, which generally lasts for about 90-120 seconds. There is a post ictal phase, which may consist of drowsiness, confusion, difficulty with speech, or muscle soreness and fatigue. Headaches are also common post ictal phenomena. Paralysis of a limb following a generalised tonic-clonic seizure with recovery from the paralysis within 24 hours is known as 'Todd's paralysis'. With the fall head injuries occur. The patient may dislocate his/her shoulder or fracture his/her thoracic vertebra during the tonic phase of the seizure. Some patients injure themselves frequently after their spells. The common injuries are head injury, burns/scalds, dental injuries, fractures and finally drowning. Many of them unfortunately belong to the small group of patients whose seizures are refractory to therapy. Sixty-five per cent of patients have no injuries, 20% have one injury, 10 % two, 5 % three or more during the course of their illness.

A few patients have a prodrome of changes in mood, or muscle twitches a day or so before the seizure. Very few state that they get an indescribable feeling before the onset of seizure. Prodrome should be differentiated from 'aura'. In Latin the word 'aura' means breeze.

The type of aura depends on the area of the brain from which it originates. The aura generally lasts for 30 seconds to a minute.

The frequency with which patients may have generalised tonic-clonic seizures varies from 2-3 per year to several fits in a day. Seizure frequency can be reduced by appropriate medication in the majority of patients. Certain situation like infection, period of severe stress and fatigue, loss of sleep and metabolic imbalance can cause an increase in frequency. Non-compliance with prescribed drug regime is the most common cause of recurrence of seizures in patients who are otherwise well controlled. Non-compliance is a fairly common problem in any large seizure clinic. This can easily be verified by obtaining level of drug or drugs in the serum.

Generalised seizures have no known cause in 60 % of cases. Positive history of seizures in near relations may be obtained. The exact genetics of this kind of seizures is still not fully worked out. It is said that if one of the parents have generalised seizure, the chance of an offspring getting a seizure increases. Head injury, perinatal anoxia, strokes, brain tumours and meningitis are some of the known causes. Arterio-venous malformations, granulomas, abscess and toxic conditions like lead encephalopathy are other conditions that cause generalised seizures.

The EEG shows a rapid train of spikes during the tonic phase of the seizure.(Fig.6.2) It changes to polyspikes and slow waves during the clonic phase, and shows diffuse slowing in the post ictal period. The post ictal changes may persist for one or two days after a seizure. An inter-ictal EEG will show abnormality in 40 % of patients. These abnormalities include generalised spikes, focal spikes and spike and waves or localised sharp slow complexes. A spike is a wave of very high frequency and sharp wave has duration of less than 70 milliseconds. The positivity of epileptiform abnormalities increase with repeated recordings, the induction of sleep, a short duration between EEG recording and the last seizure, and the use of activation procedures like sleep deprivation prior to EEG recording, hyperventilation and photic stimulation.

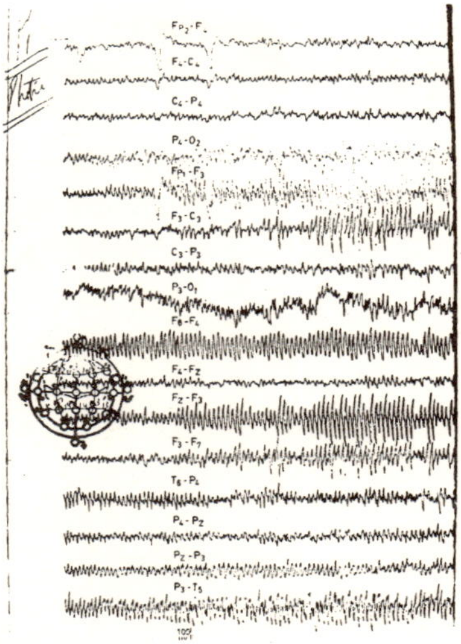

Fig 6.2. The EEG shows generalised spike discharges during tonic phase of the seizure

The diagnosis of epilepsy is primarily a clinical diagnosis and should be made on the basis of a detailed and carefully obtained history. It is of utmost important to question the patient, parents, guardians, and friends closely about the nature of the spells. When did they first begin? Did the patient have problems with seizure as a little baby? Did he have seizures with fever as a child? Did he ever lose consciousness as a result of a head injury? Did he ever have meningitis or encephalitis?

What did his first seizure consist of? Does he have a warning immediately preceding the seizure (Prodrome or aura)? Does he remember what had happened during the spell? Do his limbs jerk, does he stiffen, and does he bite his lips, cheeks or tongue? Does he pass urine or stool during the spell? Does he injure or burn himself? How long does the spell last? Does he come back to normal at once or does he have headaches, feel confused or sleepy after the seizure? Does he vomit? Do the seizures occur only during daytime, only during sleep or are they diurnal? Do they occur when he is alone? Are there any precipitating factors, like exertion, fatigue, fasting or lack of sleep? Does drinking alcohol increase the seizures? Etc.

A new case of epilepsy must be investigated with at least an EEG and when indicated a MRI brain scan, to search for a focal lesion that may be responsible for the seizure. Pseudoseizures (hysterical) may mimic generalised seizure, and the problem can be further complicated if the two may coexist in the same individual. Caution is advised before diagnosing pseudoseizures, as a rare seizure type, which either arises from the frontal lobe or supplementary motor area, may deceive the novice. When in doubt carry out 24 hour EEG telemetric recording or admit the patient and carry out video telemetric examination. In telemetric EEG examination, electrodes are applied to the patient's head and these are connected to a transmitter worn on the patient's body. The signals are then picked up by a receiver and displayed on a screen via an EEG machine. The patient is mobile in the examination room. To watch the patient a vidio camera is fixed in the room. The camera sends the pictures of the patient to the same screen on which the EEG is displayed. The clock in the camera is synchronised with the clock in the EEG machine. Hence, the observer is able to see and record simultaneously the patient's fit and its counterpart EEG. The latter will also give the advantage of closely observing the patient. The table below will help in clinically differentiating most pseudoseizures from true seizures.

Table 6.4

Differentiation Between Hysterical And Epileptic Seizure

Hysterical seizure	Epileptic seizure
Induced by emotional upsets	Needs severe stress for precipitation
Irregular periodicity as it is precipitated by minor upsets	Fairly regular periodicity
Never in sleep	Can occur during sleep
No incontinence, injury or tongue bite	One or all can occur in one of the attacks
Always in presence of people, bizarre spectacular movements.	Can occur in isolation
During unresponsiveness corneal reflex preserved	Corneal reflex absent
Eyes generally closed and resisted if opened,fists clenched tight.	Eyes rolled up and fists not clenched
Spectacular recovery with hyper-ventilation, sighing, yawning etc	Gradual recovery
Prolactin not raised	Prolactin may be raised
Telemetric EEG during attack normal	EEG during attack is abnormal

On 5th day of life at times generalised convulsions occur which has a favourable prognosis. Benign familial neonatal convulsions occur on 2nd and 3rd days of life. They have a genetic and clinical heterogeneity and the gene is located on the long arm of chromosome 20. Epilepsy occurs in 15 % of these children later. At times in infancy pyridoxine deficiency presents with convulsions. The other type of early infantile epileptic encephalopathy with poor prognosis has been described by Ohtihara and is known as Ohtihara syndrome. Infants do not survive or the ones who survive have severe handicap. It is due to dysplastic lesion.

TREATMENT : Most patients with epilepsy should continue normal activities such as schooling and working. The patient should not find himself/herself in a situation where he/she would injure the self badly if the seizure were to occur. Housewife during cooking should use a platform so that the cooking medium like gas stove is at a height. The patient should not climb on high ladder or stool. Swimming is permitted, if accompanied by a good swimmer who is aware of the disease of the patient. Patients should keep away from heavy machinery. Epileptics surprisingly have a lower accident rate than non-epileptics because they are more cautious in the workplace than their colleagues. Nothing should be done that makes the patient develop inferiority complex or lower his self esteem. Children should not be allowed to feel inferior to their peers by explanation about their disease and prescribed as far as possible twice-daily dosage of their medication, which they conveniently can take at home. Anxiety, withdrawal, somatic complaints, delinquent behaviour, aggressive behaviour, social problems and finally, attention and thought problems develop at all age groups, if proper explanation of the disease is not given to them and attention to their sleep and behavioural problems not looked into. In India, legislation regarding the rights of epileptic lags behind the industrialised countries, and this situation is badly in need of remedy. Recently, the Indian Epilepsy Association could bring about change in divorce laws. Laws regarding jobs, occupation and driving are ancient. An epileptic is not allowed to drive in India, however, in the West if the seizures are controlled and the patient is certified by a doctor and is under his direct supervision, he may be permitted to drive.

The medical therapy for generalised tonic-clonic seizures consists of choosing between any of the following drugs: Phenobarbitone, Primidone, Diphenylhydantoin sodium, Carbamazepine, Valproic acid, Sulthiame, Gabapentine, Lamotrigine, Topiramate, Oxcarbazepine, Acetazolamide, etc. Before we discuss the details of individual anticonvulsant drugs we must remember certain principles that govern their use:

a) Use drugs that you are thoroughly familiar with and use well-known drugs before trying out the less well known.
b) Use one drug and raise the dose gradually till the maximum therapeutic level is reached or signs of toxicity appear, before deciding that the drug is ineffective in seizure control.
c) Drugs with short half-life have to be given in divided doses whilst drugs with long half-life may be given in a single dose. Now with the introduction of slow release drugs, many can be given in two divided doses.
d) Time taken by a drug to reach steady state is generally five times the half-life.
e) Drugs with long half-life need a loading dose to reach steady state.
f) No drug should be discontinued suddenly as this may precipitate a status epilepticus.
g) Drug used must be specific for seizure type.

PHENOBARBITONE is one of the oldest drugs used in the treatment of epilepsy and despite many new drugs on the market, has a value in certain childhood epilepsies. It is effective in all types of partial and generalised tonic-clonic seizures. It limits high-frequency repetitive firing of action potentials by enhancing inhibitory neurotransmission by modulating GABA receptor complex. It is both safe and cheap. The cost makes it one of the commonly used drug in India even today. It is given in two divided doses in children, but may be given as a single dose in adults. A dose of 5mg/kg is prescribed in children, with adults needing about 90-120 mg per day. Injectable Phenobarb may be used in status epilepticus. The half-life of Phenonbarbital varies from 3-5 days. Adverse side effects include drowsiness, skin rash, ataxia and paradoxical hyperkinetic behaviour in children. Both Phenytoin and Valproate increase the level of Phenobarbitone in the blood while the level is diminished on administration of Ethosuximide. Action of Warfarin.is diminished when Phenobarbitone is administered simultaneously.

DIPHENYLHYDANTOIN (DPH) or Phenytoin was introduced after Phenobarbitone. It works by preventing sustained repetitive firing from extended depolarisation effected by block of voltage dependent sodium channels. It is still a first line drug for all types of partial and generalised tonic-clonic seizures. In adults it can be given as a single dose of 300 mg per day. A few patients may need a higher dose because of defective absorption or rapid metabolism. The absorption can be improved if taken with milk. The half-life of DPH varies between 21-36 hours. Patients on chronic DPH therapy should be checked for ataxia, nystagmus and gum hypertrophy. Ataxia is a sign of toxicity and indicates that the dose needs to be lowered. Drowsiness and lethargy occur at higher doses. Recently, worsening of seizures has been reported due to the drug causing encephalopathy. Phenytoin has interaction with quite a few antiepileptic drugs. The levels of Carbamazepine is either diminished or increased on simultaneous administration of Phenytoin and it is always advisable to monitor the levels of Carbamazepine when withdrawing Phenytoin. Phenytoin also diminishes the levels of Clonazepam, Ethosuximide, Felbamate, Gabapentin and Lamotrigine, while increases the levels of Phenobarbitone.

CARBAMAZEPINE is also a first line drug in all types of partial and generalised tonic-clonic seizures. Carbamazepine has a similar pharmacological anticonvulsant profile as Diphenylhydantoin. It is ideal for children, as it has neither the behavioural problems that may arise with Phenobarbital, nor the cumulative side effects of DPH such as coarsening of facial features, hirsuitism and aggravation of acne. Though, aggressiveness and temperamental changes in children are occasionally seen. Carbamazepine has a short half-life of 6-8 hours with chronic use. It should be begun at a lower dose and increased gradually to 1400-1800 mg/day. Slow release tablets are available and hence the drug can be administered twice daily. Therapeutic drug levels help in finally determining the dose. Its side effects are ataxia, dizziness, blurring of vision and diplopia. leucopenia, aplastic anaemia and thrombocytopenia have been reported as rare side effects and when evident require immediate discontinuation of the drug. Cimetidine, Erythromycin and Verapamil are known to produce clinical toxicity when administered simultaneously with Carbamazepine. Action of Warfarin is decreased on simultaneous administration with Carbamazepine. Ethosuximide, Felbamate, and Phenobarbitone diminish the levels of Carbamazepine while Phenytoin has double action, it may either increase or decrease the levels.

VALPROIC ACID is a first-line drug in all generalised epilepsies inclusive of absences, myoclonus, atonic and generalised tonic-clonic seizures. It has three different mechanism of action. It has similar action to Phenytoin and Carbamazepine on the voltage dependent sodium channel. Secondly, it reduces T-type calcium currents in primary afferent neurones. Finally it elevates whole brain GABA. Slow release tablets are available and hence, twice-daily doses suffice. The half-life of the drug is 6-8 hours. It may cause gastric irritation initially hence the drug is preferably administered after food. Major side effects include drowsiness, ataxia, weight gain and hair loss. With hair loss the dosage needs to be reduced. Hepatic dysfunction severe enough to cause death has been reported with the use of valproic acid and hence, frequent liver function tests should be done at the initiation of therapy. Platelet dysfunction is also reported due to inhibition of the arachidonate cascade. Levels of Lamotrigine, Phenobarbitone and Phenytoin are increased on simultaneous administration of Valproic acid.

PRIMIDONE causes drowsiness and ataxia, and is converted to phenobarbital in the body hence, has similar action to barbiturates like phenobarbitone. It is given in the doses of 250 mg 3-4 times a day to adults. Therapy should be initiated with 125 mg/day and gradually built up otherwise patient may develop severe drowsiness and ataxia.

LAMOTRIGINE is the newer anticonvulsant and is effective in partial and generalised seizures as well as seizures in Lennox-Gastaut syndrome. It inhibits voltage dependent sodium currents through a preferential interaction with slow-inactivated sodium channel. Thus it prevents high-frequency epileptiform discharges. It also modulates calcium conductance involved in the release of excitatory amino acids. It is excreted in breast milk and across placenta. It is effective against both simple and complex partial seizures and both primary and secondary generalised seizures. Dosage of valproic acid has to be reduced when lamotrigine is administered simultaneously. The common side effects are headaches, asthenia, erythematous, maculo-papular rash, nausea, dizziness and somnolence and sometimes insomnia. The rash usually develops, in the first 4 weeks of therapy and the drug needs to be withdrawn. In children between 2 and 12 years it is given in the dose of 0.6mg/kg of body weight (bw) and 0.15mg/kg/bw when valproic acid is being given simultaneously. Paediatric patients below 17 kg in weight should not receive the drug. In adults the dose is 5-15 mg/kg/bw (maximum 400 mg/day) and with Valproic acid 1-5 mg/kg/bw (maximum 200 mg/day). The value of monitoring plasma levels in Lamotrigine has not been established. The dose required of Lamotrigine is smaller when simultaneously administered with Valparin.

OXCARBAZEPINE is a keto analogue of Carbamazepine. Because it is similar in chemical structure to Carbamazepine, the pharmacological mechanism of action is similar. It is absorbed completely even when taken with food. The side effects are somnolence, headache, dizziness, nausea and rash. They are less as compared to Phenytoin and Carbamazepine. It also has less drug interaction than Carbamazepine. It can produce hyponatremia similar to Carbamazepine. In adults the therapy is begun at 300-600 mg/day increasing slowly to clinical effect usually up to 900-3000mg/day in two or three divided doses. In children the drug may be started at the dose of 10mg/kg/day and increased to 30mg/kg/day in divided doses. Oxcarbazepine can replace Carbamazepine and can be done abruptly. Monitoring of serum levels is generally not required. Failure of oral contraceptives has been reported during administration of Oxcarbazepine.

DPH, Carbamazepine, Oxcarbazepine, Valproic acid, and Lamotrigine raise the motor threshold over and above the actions mentioned above.

Oxcarbazepine has no interaction with other antiepileptic drugs when simultaneously administered.

GABAPENTINE is useful for treatment of partial seizures and for partial seizures becoming generalised. It is usually used as an adjunctive therapy, though it can be used in monotherapy. It is not useful for absences or myoclonus. The mechanism of its action is still not fully understood, however, it has multiple sites of action. It is usually not administered to children below 12 years. The dosage varies from 900mg/day to 3600mg/day in three divided doses. The side effects are somnolence, dizziness and fatigue.

TOPIRAMATE is another new antiepileptic drug available in India. It is absorbed rapidly, has a long duration of action and minimal interaction with other antiepileptic drugs. It is useful in refractory partial seizures with or without secondary generalisation, generalised tonic-clonic seizures and for seizures of Lennox-Gastaut syndrome specially drop attacks and for infantile spasms. The adverse effects are somnolence, dizziness, fatigue, ataxia and renal calculi. It has multiple mechanism of action, namely blockage of voltage-dependent sodium channel, potentiation of GABA, antagonises glutamate receptors and finally, inhibits erythrocyte carbonic anhydrase. An initial target dose is 200-400 mg/day in two divided doses in adults and can be raised to maximum of 800 mg/day. The ideal method would be to start at lower dose of 25-50 mg/day and increase by 25-50 mg every week in adults. In children the dose varies from 125 mg/day with body weight of 16-24 kgs, 175 mg/day for 25-35 kg body weight and 225 mg/day for children with body weight of 35-45 kg and maximum of 400 mg/kg for body weight of 45 kg and above. Phenytoin and Carbamazepine accentuates its metabolism. There is no therapeutic serum concentration for Topiramate.

The other new antiepileptics are Felbamate, Tiagabine, Vigabatrin and Zonisamide, and Levetiracetam, which are not available in India.

It is advisable to use a single drug and to increase the dose to therapeutic levels. Only when there is inadequate seizure control with an appropriate drug specific to seizure type, should another drug be added. Cases that prove resistant to adequate doses of two or more anticonvulsant drugs may need intensive study and investigated for surgery. No age is a bar to surgery. As children have larger potential for cerebral plasticity, they have a lower risk for memory loss following temporal lobectomy. Regular EEG, overnight EEG, EEG following sleep deprivation, telemetric EEG, video-telemetric EEG and EEG with special electrodes introduced extracranially such as nasal, sphenoidal or in the foramen ovale. Intracranial introduction of electrodes, such as cortical electrodes or electrodes introduced by stereotaxic surgery may also be necessary. Regular MRI with volumetric study of the amygdala and hippocampus, functional MRI, MRI spectroscopy, MRI with angiography of which one or more techniques may be necessary to localise the surgical focus. Recently, near infrared spectroscopy has been introduced to monitor cerebral oxygenation and this in turn helps to localise the focus. Single photon emission computerised tomography inter-ictal and immediate post-ictal also is of great help prior to surgery. All these procedures help to localise the epileptic focus in partial or complex partial seizures for surgery and this ultimately improves the post surgical results. Gamma knife surgery has been used for mesial temporal lobe epilepsy, which reduces invasiveness and morbidity. Surgical therapy is useful in about 10-15 % of patient with uncontrolled epilepsy. If no focus is found, in certain atonic and generalised tonic-clonic seizures corpus callosal section may be considered. In different centres, 60-80 % post-surgical improvement is mentioned. Recently, left vagal nerve stimulation is introduced for uncontrolled seizures, which are not suitable for surgery. A generator of programmed regular stimulus is introduced in the chest with coiled electrodes leading to the cervical left vagus nerve. The stimulation is given for 30 seconds every 5 minutes, 24 hours a day. Approximately 30 % of patients experience greater than 50 % reduction in seizures, and less than 10 % become seizure free. It is thought to bring about thalamic inhibition by stimulation of locus coeruleus and nucleus of solitary tract. Change in voice and hoarseness of voice has been reported. Initially, shortness of breath, bradycardia, supraventricular tachycardia, headaches and cough may occur but they disappear over a longer period of stimulation.

MYOCLONIC SEIZURES: Independent of any aetiology myoclonus is caused by hyperexcitability of cortical neurones, related to excitability cycle changes, causing hypersynchronous discharges. The centrencephalic arousal mechanism is not involved hence consciousness is preserved. Myoclonus can occur as an epileptic phenomenon or a sign in a variety of degenerative (ceroid lipofuscinosis), toxic and infectious conditions. Early myoclonic encephalopathy with non-specific cause has also been described. As an epileptic phenomenon it occurs from infancy to early childhood. Myoclonus is seen in infancy in both benign and severe forms. The benign myoclonus resolves within a month or two. The severe myoclonus is usually a symptom of various dysplastic states or malformations of the brain. In biotin deficiency, the infant is hypotonic, has sparse hair and has myoclonus. Biotin administered in 10mg. dose helps. Epilepsy with myoclonic-astatic seizure occurs in Lennox-Gastaut syndrome. As an epileptic phenomenon it occurs in young people aged 5-15 years. It consists of myoclonic jerks that occur nocturnally and may proceed to a generalised tonic-clonic seizure. The EEG may show generalised spikes or polyspikes and waves (Fig.6.3). It has a genetic background. The gene for juvenile myoclonic epilepsy with photosensitivity is located on chromosome 6p. This seizure type is known as juvenile myoclonic epilepsy and has a good prognosis. Treatment consists of Clonazepam and or Valproic acid.

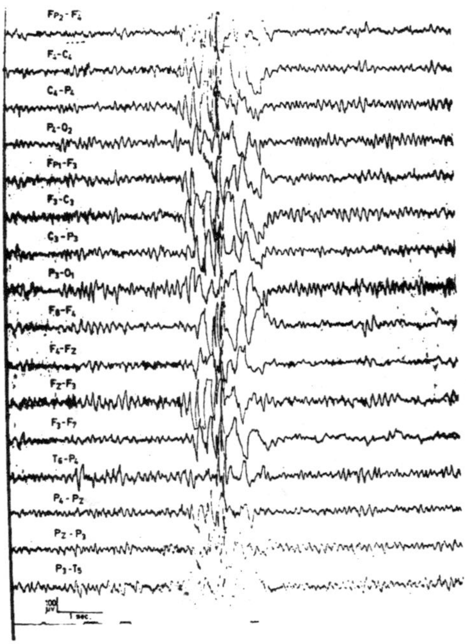

Fig 6.3 The EEG showing generalised poly-spike and wacve discharges

ATONIC SEIZURES: These seizures are difficult to control and tend to occur in individuals with diffuse brain damage. Cryptogenic variety has also been described. It is known to occur around 1-6 years of age. The child is hyperactive and has progressive cognitive dysfunction. The seizures consist of brief attacks of loss of tone, with the patient falling and injuring himself. Axial atonic seizures, tonic-clonic seizures are also known to be associated. It is designated as Lennox-Gastaut syndrome. Myoclonic seizures may be associated, it is then known as Doose syndrome. The EEG shows one to one and a half per second spike and wave discharges with slowing of the background. Valproic acid may be useful and in some cases ACTH therapy is effective. Lamotrigine, or Vigabratin or Felbamate combined with ACTH are useful. Recently vagus nerve stimulation as described earlier has been tried to control the seizures.

INFANTILE SPASMS form a part of the West's syndrome. It consists of a triad of seizures, mental retardation and hypsarhythmia on the EEG. The spasms consist of brief axial flexion or extension or both, and last less than a second. The upper half of the body flexes and the lower half extends as if in obeisance to a medieval deity (Salaam seizures). The seizures have their age of onset prior to end of the first year of life, and progress to become minor motor seizures of childhood. The symptomatic form is due to birth anoxia, phenylketonuria, tuberous sclerosis, and rarely from encephalopathy following pertussis vaccine. Cryptogenic variety is also described but is rare. The prognosis of the symptomatic variety is poor and over 90 % of the patients being severely retarded. The EEG abnormality of hypsarhythmia consists of chaotic pattern, with polyspikes and mountainous slow waves. ACTH, Prednisolone, Valproic acid, Felbamate, Zonisamide, Vigabratin and Lamotrigine all may be useful in controlling the spasms. ACTH is given in doses of 20 to 40 units daily. Prednisolone in doses of 1mg/kg/day may be used if ACTH is not available or is ineffective. Infantile spasms and Lennox-Gastaut syndrome are continuum of the same pathological process, the first arising in first few months of life and the latter between 1-4 years. Children, who develop seizures in the first few years of life, have poor prognosis, for psychomotor development.

PARTIAL SEIZURES: As stated earlier *partial seizures* are of two types the simple partial and complex partial seizures, the difference being that consciousness is preserved in the former and impaired in the latter.

ROLANDIC EPILEPSY or benign epilepsy with centro-temporal spikes: It usually occurs in young and adolescent children. The fits usually occur at night and have hemifacial motor symptomatology, like adversive movements of the head and eyes or clonic movements of face or arm. It has a genetic predisposition. Recently, it has been described with structural lesion. Carbamazepine, Oxcarbazepine and Lamotrigine, each used, as monotherapy have been found useful.

OCCIPITAL LOBE EPILEPSY: Two types of epilepsy have been described in occipital lobe involvement. The early onset benign childhood occipital seizures (EBOS) occur around 5 years of age. There are occipital spike and spike and wave discharges in EEG. Ictal vomiting and other autonomic disturbances are common. In approximately 1/3rd of cases partial status may occur. The prognosis is excellent, as most patients have 1-3 seizures in one year after which it remits. The rolandic epilepsy is more common than the occipital variety.

The late onset childhood idiopathic occipital epilepsy (LOE) occurs at 3-16 years of age with girls and boys equally affected. After 16 years of age the seizures are usually not benign and idiopathic. The seizure starts with elementary visual hallucination of small multicoloured circular patterns. They often appear in the periphery of the visual field becoming larger in the course of seizure and frequently moving horizontally to the other side. They last for few seconds to couple of minutes with sensory illusion of ocular movements and pain. There may be tonic deviation of eyes, with fluttering or repetitive eye closure. Hemiconvulsion or generalised seizure follows. Amaurosis for 3-5 minutes and migraine like headache occur post-ictally in a third of cases. Consciousness is impaired with visual symptoms, child retaining some ability to respond but unable to speak. In 10-20% the consciousness is intact and is lost during generalised seizure. EEG shows high amplitude spike and wave or sharp waves recurring rhythmically in the occipital and posterior temporal lobe of one or both hemispheres when eyes are closed. The paroxysms are frequent, brief and diurnal. MRI is mandatory and treatment with Carbamazepine has good response.

Table 6.5

Differences Between EBOS And LOE

EBOS.	LOE.
Seizure prolonged 5-30 minutes.	Short, 1-3 minutes.
No visual hallucination.	Present.
Nocturnal & infrequent. Lasts for a year.	Diurnal, frequent, often daily. 2-3 years or longer.
Excellent prognosis.	Uncertain prognosis
No medication, rectal Diazepam.	Carbamazepine.

PARTIAL SEIZURES WITH MOTOR SYMPTOMS : Any part of the body may be involved in the seizure, depending upon the side of the discharge in the motor cortex. The 'Jacksonian march' is a partial seizure in which the seizure progresses in an orderly manner, with motor activity starting in the thumb and progresses to involve the hand, the arm and later the face and half of the body. It can also begin at the angle of the mouth, spread to face and then the extremities. It can at times start at the great toe and gradually spread upwards. An adversive seizure consists of head and eyes moving to the side opposite the discharge, and sometimes progressing to a full blown tonic-clonic seizure. Occasionally aphasic seizures may be seen, the patient having difficulty with speech because of the epileptic discharge involving the speech areas. Focal seizure activity that continues for hours to months is know as 'epileptia partialis continua' of Kojenikov's epilepsy. In children it is usually due to cortical dysplasia, or encephalitis, in adults it is seen to occur in cerebro-vascular accidents, infection especially tuberculous meningitis, or viral encephalitis, Rasmussen's syndrome, cysticercosis, and hydatid cysts, subacute sclerosing panencephalitis, and metastatic tumours. Rasmussen's syndrome described in 1958 is a severe form of epilepsy with intractable motor seizures and progressive neurological deterioration. There are signs of chronic inflammatory process involving one hemisphere. If antiepileptic medication does not help, hemispherectomy may have to be resorted to.

Seizures can occur following head injury either immediately after the injury or one or two years later. The risk for post-traumatic epilepsy is higher with single temporal or frontal contusions than those without. If an EEG focus develops a month after injury, the risk becomes 4 times higher. Finally higher percentage of patients with epilepsy will show hyperintensities on MRI.

AUTOSOMAL DOMINANT FRONTAL LOBE EPILEPSY has variable age of onset. The seizures generally occur in sleep, with bizarre automatism like thrashing of legs, stereotyped sexual movements, blinking of eyes and adversive movements of head and eyes or facial myoclonus has been described recently. Abnormality in inter-ictal EEG is rare. MRI is normal. It responds to Carbamazepine. They can occur in cluster, and there is generally post-ictal confusion. It is due to mutation in neuronal nicotinic acetylcholine receptor gene on chromosome 20q13.2.

EPILEPSY WITH FRONTAL LOBE FOCUS: When the focus is in anterior frontal polar region, the patient has forced thinking, adversive movement and axial clonic jerks. With orbito-frontal focus, there are olfactory hallucinations with motor automatisms and finally with dorso-lateral frontal focus, there is tonic posturing, clonic activity, versive eye movements and speech arrest. With pre-rolandic focus, there is impaired speech, jerking of contralateral face and swallowing. And finally with frontal opercular focus, there are clonic movements of face, mastication, salivation or swallowing. When the focus extends to inferior parietal lobe, sinking, choking or nausea occurs.

AUTOSOMAL DOMINANT FAMILIAL TEMPORAL LOBE EPILEPSY: It has a familial grouping with temporal seizures described below. Can occur from 10-60 years of age. EEG and MRI are normal. The gene is on chromosome 10q. It responds to Carbamazepine.

2) PARTIAL SEIZURES WITH SOMATO-SENSORY OR SPECIAL SENSORY SYMPTOMS: Somato-sensory seizures arise from

discharges in the sensory cortex. They consist of sensation of tingling described as 'pins and needles' feeling, burning or of a feeling of numbness. Rarely a disorder of proprioception, or spatial perception occurs. Sensory seizures may also have a march like the motor seizures.

Special sensory seizures include visual seizures where hallucinations of brief duration, vary from flashes of light to vivid scenes being recalled, depending on the site of discharge. With occipito-temporo-parietal focus, the seizures consist of complex visual imagery, micropsia, and macropsia of shapes and metamorphosis of distant individuals.

Auditory hallucinations occur in epilepsy, but are common in psychotic conditions. Epileptic auditory hallucinations parallel the visual hallucinations in their elaborateness. They can vary from a single sound being repeated to a whole piece of music. Epileptic auditory hallucinations differ from those seen in psychosis, because there is no thought disorder, and the patient recalls the hallucination with a sense of detachment.

Olfactory hallucinations are generally in the form of unpleasant indescribable odours, the discharge originating in the uncus of the temporal lobe. Gustatory hallucinations parallel the sensations of taste, though commonly a metallic or bitter sensation is described. Vertiginous symptoms include a sensation of floating in space, but these seizures are rare and the reader is cautioned against calling any dizzy spell a vertiginous seizure.

Involvement of paralimbic insular cortex gives rise to viscero-motor, viscero-sensory seizures and seizures with somesthetic features.

3) COMPLEX PARTIAL SEIZURES: The complex partial seizures usually involve the temporal lobe structures. Either temporal lobe may be involved. The etiological factors vary from localised meningo-encephalitis, trauma, hamartomas and tumours, and following febrile seizures. It can arise at any time of life from 3-35 years of age. It is more predominant in males than females. Benign complex partial seizures with automatism have been described in children of 2-3 years of age. The psychic symptoms include dysamnesic symptoms such as deja vu, a feeling of familiarity with an unfamiliar situation,

and jamais-vu where the patient feels strange in very familiar surroundings. Cognitive disturbances including dreamy states, distortion of time sense and feelings of depersonalisation (autoscopy) may occur.

Seizures with affective symptomatology include those with fear, pleasure, anger, and depression. These occur in less than 5 per cent of patients. Fear is intense, stark and brief. Pleasure includes a feeling of serenity and well-being, though ecstatic states have been described. Anger is unprovoked, non-directive, and dissipates rapidly. Patient is resistant to restrain. The patient has no memory for his behaviour. 10-30 % can arise from extra-temporal origin. Directive violence has not been shown to be of epileptic origin, in fact violent acts occur very rarely with complex partial seizures, and are fragmentary in nature. Depression can be profound and can last for days. It frequently culminates in a generalised tonic-clonic seizure.

Gelastic seizure consists of inappropriate laughter, the laugh being hollow, the facial expression unchanged and the patient unaware later of his action. There are multiple sites of origin of gelastic seizure but is commonly seen with hamartoma of the hypothalamus occasionally with precocious puberty. It can be mixed with other seizure types. EEG and SPECT help in localisation. Radio-frequency thermocoagulation of the hamartoma may be carried out. When the complex partial seizure arises in amygdala, patient gets a feeling of Déjà vu, a cephalic sensation or a warm sensation which is non-describable strange sensation and sensation of fear.

With deep sylvian or opercular focus, there may be gustatory hallucinations, nausea, and epigastric sensation of something mounting up and feeling of butterflies and lightness. Focus in the superior temporal gyrus produces auditory hallucinations of simple sounds or complex language.

When the complex partial seizure arises in the dominant temporal lobe, there is more pertinent interruption of contact with the surroundings and the vocalisation is of sound only. There may be aphasia, amnesia and prolonged post ictal dysphasic deficit. On the other hand if the seizure arises from the non-dominant temporal lobe, the seizure is short with ictal articulate speech; automatism with preserved consciousness or responsiveness. There is usually a quick recovery.

The most common type of complex partial seizure is the 'psychomotor' variety. It consists of three phases: the first phase begins with a non-specific aura. The aura usually lasts for few seconds to a minute. The aura is a feeling described by patients just prior to the seizure. It may consist of epigastric sensation, a 'funny feeling' in the head, fear or feeling of unreality. Then follows a phase of total unresponsiveness, the patient being immobile with a vacant stare, a facial grimace and head turning often herald the seizure. If examined at this stage, the pupils are dilated and non-reactive to light, but react in the later phase of the seizure. The head and eye deviation is of two types, the early and late. With early deviation the seizure origin may be in the ipsilateral temporal lobe, while late head turning precludes to generalisation.

The second phase consists of automatism. Automatism in a complex partial seizure may be stereotyped, consisting of aimless movements such as lip licking, lip smacking are detected in the majority. The fumbling, picking, brushing movements of the hands are not of definitive localising value but are seen mostly with ipsilateral focus. The dystonic movements of the arms and lower extremities localise the focus to contralateral temporal lobe in the majority. Sometimes patient may walk about and may have elaborate semipurposeful co-ordinated movements, or utter a few words, which though recognisable are irrelevant to the situation. The patient is amnesiac for these events. The final phase is the longest and can last up to 15 minutes. The patient is confused and gradually recovers from the seizure. Reactive automatism occurs in some patients in the post ictal period.

It is important to differentiate partial complex seizures from absences. The presence of an aura, the longer duration, the complex automatism and gradual return to normal consciousness help differentiate between the two.

SIMPLE PARTIAL SEIZURES are commonly focal motor in character, though any of the above mentioned varieties may occur, but the seizure should only be classified as simple partial if consciousness remains unimpaired through out the seizure.

Illusions and autonomic symptoms may rarely occur as partial seizures.

The diagnosis of partial seizures is sometimes difficult and may require prolonged EEG monitoring with video telemetry. A carefully taken history will suffice in the all but a very small number of patients. The EEG shows localised spikes or sharp waves in an inter-ictal recording. Use of nasopharyngeal, sphenoidal or foramen ovale electrodes, enhances the likelihood of detecting a fronto-temporal focus. EEG following overnight sleep deprivation also increases the chances of detecting the abnormal focus. Focal motor seizures in children are generally not indicative of focal brain pathology, except Tuberous sclerosis, arachnoid cyst, dysplasia in some and Rasmussen's encephalitis in a rare case. In older patients there is one in ten chance of finding a tumour, cyst, local or generalised atrophy following head injury, arterio-venous malformation or infarct. Recently, there has been spate of reports of single enhancing ring lesion on CAT scan examination, which may disappear after anticonvulsive treatment, which is generally due to cysticercosis. If it persists for more than three weeks, than there is a possibility that the lesion is a tuberculoma. Rarely the lesion is due to focal granulomatous encephalitis.

The treatment of partial seizures is similar to that of generalised tonic-clonic seizure except that Valproic acid is unlikely to be of value. DPH, Carbamazepine, Oxcarbazepine, Lamotrigin and Topiramate are the most useful drugs in these seizures. Patients who do not respond to adequate medical therapy should be offered surgical therapy. Partial seizures arising from posterior temporal, parieto-temporal and occipital regions are a substantial problem both medically and surgically. The seizure may have diffuse onset involving large cortical area, or may have a focal onset with rapid spread to association areas via projection fibres. Hence, there is difficulty in localisation of the focus. The surgical outcome also depends on the technique (Topectomy, subpial transaction and lobectomies), and complete resection of the epileptic focus. Surgery in the frontal lobe area has better prognosis. Fifty per cent derive benefit from occipital lobe surgery while only 25 to 35 % derive benefit from posterior temporal parieto-temporal surgery. Temporal lobectomy is to be considered for complex partial seizures. It is important to localise from which temporal lobe does the seizure originate. Initially, clinical observation with video-telemetric EEG examination should be carried out. The next investigation is MRI as hippocampal sclerosis is the most common pathology. On MRI there is increased hippocampal T2 signal with decreased signal on T1 and hippocampal atrophy. The next investigation is SPECT both inter-ictal and post-ictal. Hypo-perfusion in the inter-ictal phase and hyper-perfusion in the post ictal phase is noted. Unfortunately, surgical therapy is available and indicated in only a small number of patients with intractable seizures. Twenty-five per cent of patients derive good benefit and are seizure free, 40 % have reduced number of seizures and 35 % have poor outcome. Best results with unitemporal inter-ictal spikes and unilateral mesial temporal sclerosis on MRI. Earlier the onset worst is the prognosis. It is said that patients having normal inter-ictal EEG have better prognosis while patients with anterior or mid-temporal spikes do not fare as well. Patients with lateral cortical lesions fair better than patients do with hippocampal sclerosis on surgery.

Rare types of partial seizures include seizures from supplementary motor area. During a seizure the head and eyes turn to one side, the contralateral arm is raised and abducted and the leg may be extended. Autonomic disturbance such as palpitations and a flushing sensation has also been reported.

Landau-Kleffner syndrome occurs at the age of 2-7 years in previously healthy children. The child loses language function for a week or months. The symptoms recover with antiepileptic medication or sometimes spontaneously within 2 years. More than 2/3rd have permanent language dysfunction. Scalp EEG shows high amplitude mid temporal spikes and spike and waves. Sound also induces spikes. Antiepileptic medication like Carbamazepine, Lamotrigine is recommended. In intractable cases steroids or intravenous immunoglobulins may be tried.

EPILEPSY CHARACTERISED BY DIFFERENT MODES OF STIMULATIONS:

READING EPILEPSY: The seizures are precipitated by reading aloud and are independent of the text that is being read. There is perioral reflex myoclonus. It has been shown that there is hypoperfusion in the temporal lobe during the ictus. Perioral reflex myoclonus can also occur in generalised and partial seizures.

HOT WATER EPILEPSY: This has been described from South India but has been known to occur all over the country. The complex partial seizure occurs on pouring hot water over the head during a bath. Patient also gets seizures even without a bath. The complex partial seizure may end in a generalised seizure.

SEIZURES OCCURRING ON PHOTIC STIMULATION: Generally myoclonus and /or generalised seizures occur on intermittent photic stimulation, either during an EEG recording or with flashing and fluctuating lights. It is usually seen in 7-19 year age group and remits in 25 % after second decade. It can also occur while driving, during the day with strong sunlight, along a road lined with trees. Some patients get fits while watching television or playing video games. Optical filters reduce level of photic stimulation of televised images and thereby prevent photosensitive seizures. It is suggested that, it may have a genetic basis.

Idiopathic photosensitive occipital epilepsy occurs on watching television, playing video games or on other photic triggers. Multicoloured circular visual hallucinations often associated with blindness, tonic deviation of eyes with epigastric discomfort and vomiting has been described in this type seizures. Headache and generalised seizure may follow. The seizure lasts for 2-5 minutes. The prognosis is uncertain. The inter-ictal EEG shows either spontaneous or photic induced occipital spikes. Centro-temporal spikes may co-exist.

MUSICOGENIC EPILEPSY: Generally precipitated by hearing any type of music and has a right superior temporal lobe onset.

STATUS EPILEPTICUS

Though previously defined as a state in which there is no recovery from consciousness between seizures, it is now defined as a condition where clinical or electrical seizure activity lasts for at least thirty minutes, whether or not consciousness is impaired. The classification of status epilepticus is given below:

Table 6.6

Types of Status Epilepticus

Convulsive status	Nonconvulsive status
a) Primary generalised major motor status i. Tonic-clonic status ii. Myoclonic status	a) Spike-wave stupor or Absence status
b) Partial or focal status i. Focal motor status (Jacksonian status) ii. Epilepsia partialis continua	a) Complex partial status or psychomotor status
c) Generalised major motor with partial onset i. Adversive onset ii. Partial motor onset	

We shall restrict our discussion to major motor status, as it is the most common and most serious form of status. Brief discussion of absence status and partial complex status are included so that the reader is aware of these entities when he examines a case of prolonged altered consciousness.

<u>MAJOR MOTOR STATUS EPILEPTICUS</u>: 60 to 80 % of cases have a focal onset, either adversive or partial motor. The clonic component of the seizure progressively decreases until only tonic seizures occur. Status is not a part of the natural history of epilepsy; therefore the cause of the status must be looked for. Infection, metabolic imbalance, electrolyte disturbance, and withdrawal from alcohol are important causes of status. Sudden discontinuation of anticonvulsant medication is a common cause of status. Sometimes a new neurological condition such as the occurrence of a subdural haematoma or the presence of a neoplasm leads to a status. Degenerative conditions like Lafora body disease, Kuf's disease or tuberous sclerosis are rare causes of status.

The average duration of a status is nearly 3 hours. The mortality varies between 10 to 15 %. Status is a neurological emergency that requires prompt attention. Permanent brain damage occurs if the status lasts for more than an hour. The Purkinje cells of the cerebellum, layers 3, 5 and 6 of the cerebral cortex, and Sommer's sector of the hippocampus suffer the most. If adequate oxygenation is maintained through out the status, the degree of neuronal loss is reduced and is restricted to hippocampus.

The aims of therapy in status are:

1. To try and stop the status as soon as possible preferably within thirty minutes.
2. To prevent the recurrence of seizure activity.
3. To maintain adequate oxygenation and blood pressure.
4. To correct any metabolic or electrolyte imbalance, and to search for the cause of infection.

A protocol can be followed in the management of status as follows:

Maintain an airway, and if necessary intubate the patient. Insert an intragastric tube and pass a urinary Foley's catheter. 50 cc. of 50% glucose may be given intravenously or 100 cc of intravenous mannitol, after drawing the blood for glucose, electrolytes, ketones, renal and liver function tests, and blood culture if an infection is suspected and finally serum for anti-convulsant drug levels. If there is history of diabetes, glucose and mannitol may be withheld.

Start an intravenous drip, and inject 10 mg of Diazepam (or 2mg per kg.) no faster than 2 mg per minute. The drug reaches the brain in 10 seconds and stops the seizure in nearly 70 per cent of patients with status. Diazepam concentration in the brain drops drastically in twenty minutes, therefore a drug that prevents further seizures has to be given next. For intravenous use DPH and Valproic acid are available. Under ECG and blood pressure control, one gram of intravenous DPH may be given, at the rate of 50 mg per minute as a loading dose. If monitoring facilities are not available, infusion of Valproic acid 20-40 mg/kg, diluted 1:1 may be safer drug to administer over 1 to 5 minutes. If neither is possible, syrup Dilantin, 2 teaspoonful (200 mg DPH) may be given every two hours for five doses. Phenobarbitone is given in doses of 300 to 400 mg (or 20 mg/kg) if the status is not controlled with DPH or Valproic acid.

Paraldehyde in a dose of 10 ml, 5 ml in each buttock, is very useful in many cases of intractable status. A Diazepam drip, with 100 mg of diazepam diluted in 500 ml of 5% glucose, given at the rate of 40 ml per hour is recommended in those cases that do not respond to the measures outlined above. Intravenous Thiopental in a dose of 0.5 to 1 gm in 500 ml of normal saline may be used. The rate of infusion is titrated to maintain the patient in light anaesthesia. The thiopental drip is only recommended in the most severe cases, and anaesthesiology supervision is recommended. Finally, if for any reason, intravenous route for administration of drugs is not available, Midazolam in the dose of .05 to 2 mg/kg may be given intramuscularly. In children it can be administered intranasally in the same dosage.

CONTINUOUS SPIKE AND WAVE ACTIVITY DURING SLOW WAVE SLEEP: It represents an EEG pattern common to a number of different widely varying clinical types of epilepsy. The epilepsy may be cryptogenic or symptomatic. It can be called a subclinical electrical status induced by sleep in children. It occurs around 5 -10 years of age equally in boys and girls. It usually disappears after 12 years of age. Later in awake stage focal or multifocal EEG abnormality may persist.

NON-CONVULSIVE STATUS

ABSENCE STATUS: It can last from hours to days, the patient having a history of absences, or generalised tonic-clonic seizures. Stress or trauma precipitates the status. The patient appears slow and has paucity of speech. The patient may carry out daily activities such as brushing teeth etc., but does not interact with the environment normally and appears withdrawn. Myoclonic twitches may occur. The diagnosis is made on EEG, which shows generalised spike and waves. Intravenous Diazepam breaks the status both clinically and electrically. High dose of Valproic acid is used on a chronic basis.

COMPLEX PARTIAL STATUS :It consists of two phases that alternate in cyclical manner, a phase of total unresponsiveness with speech arrest and stereotyped automatism and a phase of partial responsiveness with partial speech and quasi-purposeful automatism similar to that of major motor status. It is treated in a similar manner as the partial status epilepticus.

CHAPTER VII CEREBRO-VASCULAR DISEASE

A large population develops stroke as the age advances. The incidence of stroke and the mortality due to stroke is high. The exact figures of annual incidence, prevalence, morbidity and mortality, for the entire Indian subcontinent are not available. However, from the few studies done in various regions of the country, the crude prevalence rate is around 200 per 100,000 populations. The figures are highest in the Parsi community (843/100,000). In the developed countries this figure is around 100-180 per 100,000. In India approximately 2 % of all hospital admissions are of patients with stroke of which a small percentage is in the younger patients below the age of 40 years. The incidence of stroke increases with increasing age. Strokes are more common in males than females. Every year about 500,000 Americans experience a new stroke or a recurrent stroke. Of these, about a third die and of the remaining 30% require some assistance, 20 % require assistance for ambulating, and remaining 20 % need institutional care.

We cannot alter the gender, the age, the family history or the genetics. The presence of Marfan's syndrome, Ehler-Danlos syndrome, Sturge-Weber disease, atrial myxoma, hereditary cardiomyopathy and cardiac conduction disorders, deficiency of protein C and S, presence of Willebrand's factor, antithrombin III with increased blood viscosity, mitochondrial disorders and Fabry's disease are just a few genetic factors in the causation of stroke. However, there are a large number of causative factors for stroke, which can be medically attended to. Uncontrolled diabetes, with retinopathy and autonomic neuropathy, increases the mortality and morbidity by 2 to 4 folds. Hypertension is present in more than a half of patients admitted with stroke, which if detected in time and treated will prevent stroke. Smoking and tobacco chewing is common in India, and is well known that tobacco increases both cardio-vascular and cerebro-vascular accidents. High cholesterol with increased low-density cholesterol and alpha lipoprotein, leading to dyslipidemia, again is a major factor in the causation of stroke. There is an inverse relationship between high-density lipoprotein and cerebro-vascular disease. Low levels of high-density lipoproteins are associated with increased risk of rupture of atherosclerotic plaques. High triglyceride levels in coronary heart disease predict stroke and TIA. This relationship is independent of age, sex, patient characteristic and level of cholesterol fractions. Though moderate alcohol consumption (two drinks or less a day) is helpful in prevention of strokes, and is associated with lesser occurrence of white matter abnormalities and infarcts of vascular origin, seen on MRI. Chronic alcohol dependence and binge drinking increases the incidence of subclinical atherosclerosis and strokes. Oral contraceptives, tablets enhancing male erectile function, obesity, elevated homocysteinuria due to folate deficiency, anaemia, elevated anticardiolipin antibodies, increased fibrinogen are other factors increasing the incidence of stroke. Patients with valvular dysfunctions due to rheumatic fever and other causes, cardiomyopathies, cardiac conduction defects and bacterial endocarditis are cardiac causative factors of stroke. Non-valvular atrial fibrillation present in almost 60-70 per cent of elderly between the ages of 65 and 85 years is an important factor in the causation of stroke.

Table 7.1

Non-Atherosclerotic Causes Of Stroke

Cardiac	Prosthetic valves, clots, tumours, air and fat embolism, rhythm changes
Haematological	Polycythemia, sickle cell disease, lymphoproliferative diseases, thrombotic thrombocytopenic purpura, procoagulant states, anticardiolipin antibody syndrome
Vascular-arterial	Vasospasm, trauma, fibromuscular dysplasia, dissection, post radiation damage, atreritis due to tuberculosis, syphilis and collagen diseases
Vascular -venous	Venous sinus thrombosis, procoagulant states

The important factor in causation of thrombosis or embolism is the presence of atherosclerosis. Atherosclerotic lesion starts with accumulation of low-density lipoprotein (LDL) in the blood vessel. This LDL gets oxidised and starts the chain of events, which lead to formation of an atherosclerotic plaque. The LDL initially accumulates in the extracellular subendothelial space of the arteries. The LDL is then modified by oxidation. This oxidised LDL stimulates the resident vascular cells to produce monocyte chemotactic protein. This protein in turn stimulates monocytes to acquire the function of macrophages and also stimulates monocytes to bind to the vascular endothelial cells. A colony of granulocytes and macrophages develop. The macrophages massively ingest cholesterol from oxidised LDL and turn into foam cells. The monocytes get trapped in subendothelial space as oxidised LDL inhibits their egress from the arterial wall. The oxidised LDL is cytotoxic to these macrophages and promotes liberation of lipids and liposomal enzymes into the intimal extracellular space. This in turn enhances the progression of atherosclerosis and plaque formation. Autoantibodies to oxidised LDL develop and it is found that plasma concentration of immunoreactive antibodies to oxidised LDL is higher after an acute myocardial infarct. The development of plaque formation is not related to age. The plaque ultimately ruptures which leads to vasoconstriction and thrombosis. The mechanism that causes this rupture is incompletely understood. Local inflammation due to abundant macrophages and T-cells, which degrade the extra-cellular matrix, has been considered as one of the mechanism responsible for the plaque rupture. The necrotic debris from the ruptured plaque stimulates release of proteolytic enzymes from necrotic macrophages, which alter the structural integrity of the fibrous cap covering the plaque leading to ulcer formation.

Normally vascular endothelium prevents adhesion of leukocytes and platelets to the inner vascular surface by release of endothelial derived Nitrous Oxide (NO). The oxidised LDL prevents the release of NO in normal arteries. There is also direct inactivation NO by lipid peroxidation products of oxidised LDL. Increased production of super oxide by the vascular endothelium also leads to loss of activation of NO. Physiological inactivation of NO leads to adhesion of platelets, this is yet another factor for causation of thrombosis, embolism and transient ischemic episodes.

Finally, proliferation of the smooth muscle cells leads to vascular stenosis, near the plaque.

In summary, increased monocyte adhesion, with increased foam cell formation, leading to increased cyto-toxicity and increased vascular dysfunction leads to atherogenesis. This ultimately results in thrombo-embolism.

The arterial wall of the intracranial arteries is made up of three layers. The outer layer called the adventitia, the middle layer called the media and the inner layer is called the intima, which is made of endothelial cells. This normally provides a non-thrombotic surface. The cerebral arteries lack the internal elastic lamina. The arterioles contain the smooth muscle cells but the capillaries are made up of only thin layer of endothelial cells. The nutrients and the metabolites diffuse through the capillaries. Veins have a fragile muscle cell wall.

Once the artery is occluded, there is reduced blood supply to microcirculation. This leads to impairment of brain energy metabolism by loss of aerobic glycolysis. There is migration of sodium and calcium ions into the cells, leading to neuronal swelling, later hyperchromatism, pyknosis, chromatolysis and finally shrinkage of the cell. There is also swelling and fragmentation of astrocytes and endothelial cells. There is release of excito-toxic neurotransmitters. There is also elevation of lactate levels with production of local acidosis. There is over activation of lipases and proteases leading to cell death. The central area thus becomes necrotic. Neutrophils invade the necrotic area as early as within 4 hours and is abundant by 36 hours. Oedema occurs within and around the infarct. Within 48 hours microcytes proliferate ingest the myelin breakdown products and form macrophages. Ultimately the area of necrosis is absorbed and cavitation occurs. The glia and fibrovascular structure line the wall. Neovascularisation due to proliferation of capillaries with increased prominence of existing capillaries takes place. In a large infarct there are three distinct zones. As described earlier, there is inner area of coagulation necrosis, with central zone of vacuolated neuropil and leukocyte infiltration. The second zone consists of swollen area with oedema and thickened capillaries. The outer marginal area consists of hyperplastic astrocytes, with variable changes in nuclear staining.

In complete stroke, the suppression of electrical activity occurs within 12-15 seconds. The synaptic transmission stops by 2-4 minutes and total inhibition of all electrical activity occurs after 4-6 minutes. The normal blood flow in normal individual is approximately 50-55 ml/100gm/minute. When the flow diminishes to 18ml/100gm/minute the brain loses electrical function, but on restoration of the flow, the function can recover. On the other hand if the flow is reduced to 8ml/100gm/minute, the membrane failure occurs leading to cell death. In the area of ischemic penumbra, where the flow rate is between the two rates mentioned above, some neurones become functionally silent but are structurally intact and are salvageable. The ischemic penumbra depends on the size of the vessel and availability of collateral blood supply.

The infarct is usually wedge shaped in the centre of the arterial territory with the occlusion of the main artery. When carotid artery is involved the infarct is multilobar with severe oedema, with flattening of the gyri and obliteration of the sulci. Lacunar infarcts occur due to involvement of the smaller vessel. The size of lacune is around 1.5 cm diameter or less. It is usually due to embolus and is generally at the junction of the cortex and white matter. They can either be single or multiple and may be either symptomatic or asymptomatic. The most common ones produce motor hemiparesis, with a lesion in internal capsule, corona radiata or basis pontis. The second variety is ataxic hemiparesis due to a lesion in the posterior limb of the internal capsule or basis pontis. In the sensory motor stroke due to a lacunar infarct, the lesion is in the internal capsule, thalamus or is striato-capsular. The pure sensory stroke is due to a lesion in ventro-posterior parietal lobe or thalamus. Finally, the clumsy hand dysarthria syndrome is due to a lesion in the deep areas of the pons.

Following an infarct, the platelet count and its adhesiveness are increased. The ESR is raised. Plasma fibrinogen is increased with diminution in fibrinolytic activity. The beta lipoproteins and triglycerides also show a rise. In larger infarct, the CSF pressure rises with increased in CSF proteins. The CAT scan helps differentiate between haemorrhage and infarct. The perfusion scan can help to work out the size of the infarct and thereby the prognosis. In middle cerebral artery thrombosis, at times the vessel appears prominent on CAT scan. This generally indicates a poor prognosis. From day 5 onwards, the T1 weighted images on MRI show an isointense lesion, while on T2 the infarct is hyperintense. The diffusion pictures show hyperintesity early. From 5 - 15 days the infarcted area is hyperintense on both T1 and T2 weighted images

The middle cerebral artery arises at the bifurcation of the internal carotid artery above the cavernous sinus. The artery then enters the Sylvian fissure where it divides into three branches, the precentral, posterior parietal and posterior temporal branches. Also given off in the Sylvian fissure are six to ten thin penetrating vessels known as lenticulo-striate branches that supply the basal ganglia, the internal capsule and the optic radiation.

It is noted that 80% of strokes occur in the carotid or anterior circulation and 20% in the posterior circulation that is vertebro-basilar territory. Transient ischemic episodes (TIA) also occur with the same frequency in each territory. They are due to sudden, temporary, focal, non-marching neurological deficit. The last part is important as focal fits generally have a march. The attack usually lasts for 5-20 minutes. In these attacks, ischemia may occur either in retina, cochlea or brain or brain stem. There is generally a complete recovery. Headache is a common symptom occurring with TIA. They occur due to severe arterial stenosis and ulcerated plaques with formation of platelet thrombi and their release in the distal circulation. 10-30 % may be due to release of thrombi from the heart. Prolapsed mitral valve can also cause TIA. Increased adhesiveness of the platelet, polycythemia and hyper-coagulable states are other factors known to cause TIA. The treatment consists of administration either of, aspirin and/or Clopidrogel and /or Dypiramidol. Endarterectomy of the carotid or insertion of a stent in the carotid is advised if the stenotic lesion involves more than 70 % of the arterial lumen.

It is very important to note that bilateral shifting motor or sensory deficit, complete or partial loss of vision in both homonymous fields, peri-oral numbness, isolated diplopia, vertigo, dysarthria or dysphagia should not be considered TIA unless they occur in combination with one another or with any other symptom.

It will not be out of place to mention subclavian steal syndrome, at this juncture. This is usually due to stenosis or occlusion of the subclavian artery proximal to the origin of vertebral artery. Left side involvement is frequent. Symptoms of brain stem ischemia develop due to reversal of flow in the vertebral artery on exercising the arm supplied by the stenosed subclavian artery. The stealing of blood occurs from the vertebral artery due to excess demand by the exercised arm, which is not met with by the stenosed subclavian artery. There is reduced blood pressure with delayed radial pulse in the affected arm.

The drop attacks are thought to be due to sudden ischemia of the cortico-spinal tract or reticular formation in the vertebro-basilar territory. They are also known to occur with high cervical and foramen magnum lesions. Sudden loss of tone in akinetic seizures can lead to drop attacks.

Finally, during the attack of a transient global amnesia there is reversible anterograde and retrograde memory loss with total amnesia of event. There is inability to learn and retain newly acquired information and hence, the patient keeps on asking the same question repeatedly. Patient remains alert, retains personal identity, can carry on complex activity and is without motor or sensory impairment. These attacks occur commonly after the age of 50 and are commoner in males. They usually last for 3-6 hours but seldom longer then 12 hours. Nothing is known about their causation except that they may be similar in aetiology to migraine.

OCCLUSION OF THE MAIN TRUNK OF THE CAROTID ARTERY causes a large area of infarction with involvement of multiple lobes and massive oedema of the affected hemisphere. The oedema may be so severe that it may cause pressure on the brain stem and lead to coma. Occlusion of the middle cerebral artery on the dominant side produces global aphasia, and apraxia whilst non-dominant lesion produces loss of body image on the contralateral side and denial of the existence of the left side of the body. There is profound flaccid hemiplegia; the arm being more affected than the leg. Hemianaesthesia and a complete hemianopia also occur in this most devastating stroke. Death occurs if a pressure cone forms and gives rise to severe brain stem compression. Death can also occur later if the infarct transforms into a haemorrhagic variety.

When carotid artery is occluded in young children, for example, following infections of throat, leash of vessel at the base of the brain open up. The angiographic picture of this resembles a cloud known as Moyamoya in Japanese language. The patient usually presents with strokes or convulsions and later may present with subarachnoid haemorrhage.

Recently, a condition called CADASIL – cerebral autosomal dominant arteriopathy with subcortical infarcts and leukoencephalopathy, has been described. The clinical picture is with attacks of migraine with aura, mood disturbances, and recurrent subcortical strokes and step wise or progressive dementia. There is mutation of Notch 3 gene on chromosome 19.

OCCLUSION OF THE LENTICULO-STRIATE BRANCHES usually leads to a pure motor hemiplegia with flaccidity occurring only fleetingly in the early stage of the disease. Tone begins to recover in a few hours and exaggerated reflexes and an extensor plantar response are observed. Speech may be slurred due to facial weakness, but there is no aphasia. Power recovers gradually and the patient is left with the typical hemiplegic posture and gait. Lacunar infarcts in the internal capsule and this lesion are the commonest varieties of stroke and they have a good prognosis for recovery.

LESIONS ON THE DOMINANT SIDE:

OCCLUSION OF THE PRECENTRAL BRANCH causes paralysis of the face and arm (facio-brachial lesion), and a total inability to speak; though the ability to comprehend spoken speech is retained. The patient is unable to write and appears markedly frustrated by the speech deficit. Speech therapy may help to some extent. Patient learns few words, by which he is able to communicate.

OCCLUSION OF THE CENTRAL BRANCH leads to weakness of the face and arm, with minimal non-fluent aphasia.

OCCLUSION OF THE POSTERIOR PARIETAL BRANCH produces fluent aphasia with difficulty in comprehending spoken speech. A mild hemiparesis and cortical sensory loss with 'inattention' occurs. Sensory inattention is the ignoring of one side on bilateral simultaneous stimulation. Sensory signs may be difficult to elicit in some patients because of problem with communication.

NON-DOMINANT HEMISPHERE LESION:

OCCLUSION OF THE PRECENTRAL AND CENTRAL BRANCHES leads to facial and arm weakness only.

OCCLUSION OF THE POSTERIOR PARIETAL AND SUPERIOR TEMPORAL BRANCHES lead to dressing apraxia and loss of recognition of faces (prosopagnosia). There is also loss of topographical memories. Dressing apraxia results in the patient sometimes putting his arms through one sleeve of his shirt and being unaware that he has forgotten the other sleeve. Prosapognosia leaves him unable to recognise the faces of relatives, but he can recognise them by voice. Loss of topographical memory results in the patient being lost in his own home and not finding his way around his neighbourhood. Cortical sensory loss and minimal hemiparesis may also occur as a result of vascular occlusion.

OCCLUSION OF THE ANTERIOR CEREBRAL ARTERY produces greater weakness in the leg due to involvement of the parasagittal area. Cortical sensation in the weak limb may be affected. The other features of frontal lobe involvement are memory loss, cognitive impairment, and loss of social sense and euphoria. Voluntary sudden movement of the eyes in the contralateral direction may be affected. There may be a grasp reflex on examination. In lesion on dominant side if Broca's area is affected, fluent speech may be lost.

OCCLUSION OF THE POSTERIOR CIRCULATION

Occlusion of the top of the basilar artery produces lesions in the mid-brain, thalamus, portion of the temporal lobe and occipital lobe. The patient is drowsy, has hallucinations of human beings, animals and insects moving around (peduncular hallucinosis), has impairment of memory, and may have an agitated delirium. Has bilateral paresis of the upward or downward gaze, with impaired convergence, skew deviation and oscillatory eye movements. Patient may also have hemianopia or cortical blindness. The pupils are both small and reactive or are fixed in mid-position.

Lesions in the pons that involve the vestibular nuclei cause vertigo due to involvement of the posterior inferior cerebellar artery.

Associated with this is the lesion in the lateral medulla, with resulting difficulty in swallowing, Horner's syndrome and cerebellar signs ipsilaterally. Facial sensation is lost on the same side while there is loss of sensation on the opposite side of the body. This is known as Wallenburg's syndrome. The Millard-Gubler syndrome consists of sixth nerve palsy and facial palsy on the side of the lesion with a contralateral hemiplegia. Foville's syndrome is similar to Millard-Gubler syndrome except that conjugate gaze palsy replaces the sixth nerve palsy. A lesion of the medial medulla causes ipsilateral paralysis of the muscles of the tongue, and a contralateral hemiplegia that spares the face. Loss of postural sensibility also occurs. Locked-in state occurs with occlusion of the main vertebral artery causing an infarct of the brain stem below the third nerve nucleus, leading to total quadruparesis but sparing the reticular formation. Patient is awake, able to hear but unable to phonate and carries out conversation by movement of the eyes.

Table 7.2

Neurological Deficits Resulting From Lesions Of Pyramidal Tracts At Different Levels

Cortical lesion	Flaccid hemiplegia with focal convulsion and other cortical signs such as aphasia, apraxia, etc
Internal capsule	Spastic hemiplegia with or without sensory involvement and/or hemianopia
Upper mid-brain lesion	Superior gaze palsy with contralateral hemiplegia (Weber's syndrome), Coarse tremors with contralateral hemiplegia (Benedict's syndrome)
Pons	Vertigo at onset, 6th and/or 7th nerve with contralateral hemiplegia (Millard-Gubler syndrome). Conjugate gaze palsy with contralateral hemiplegia (Foville's syndrome)
Medial medulla	Ipsilateral tongue with contralateral hemiplegia and posterior column involvement
Lateral medulla	Palatal weakness, Horner's syndrome ipsilateral facial sensory loss, ipsilateral cerebellar signs and contralateral hemianaesthesia (Wallenberg's syndrome).
Upper cervical cord	Spastic hemiplegia without cranial nerve involvement

In vast majority of cases with vascular pathology, the lesion is either due to embolism, thrombosis or haemorrhage. This usually affects as stated earlier, either the carotid or vertebral system. Embolic lesion begins suddenly and may even present as a focal seizure. There may be history of TIA. Emboli can arise from the heart, as in mitral stenosis, mitral valve prolapse, auricular fibrillation, myocardial infarction with clots in the heart and subacute bacterial endocarditis. Emboli have also been described in atrial myxoma. Emboli may also arise in merentic thrombi on cardiac valves in patients with carcinoma. Polycythemia is a rare cause of TIA. Common sources of emboli however, are debris from ulcerative plaques of atherosclerosis in the large arteries supplying the brain. Atherosclerotic plaques tend to occur at the bifurcation of the major arteries such as carotid. Emboli are said to occur more commonly in the territory of vertebral artery. Ischemic lesions those are secondary to atheroma, syphilis or tuberculous arteritis result in thrombosis. Thrombosis comes on gradually, most commonly while the patient is asleep. Hypertension, diabetes, obesity and hyperlipidemia are the major risk factors as stated earlier.

Table 7.3

Clues To Pathophysiological Process

THROMBOSIS	EMBOLISM	HAEMORRHAGE
Older age	Young age	Begins during activity
Previous TIAs	Valvular heart disease	Headache
Gradual onset	Very acute onset	Gradual sensorium affectation
Begins in quiet period	Convulsion at onset	Convulsions
Progression over hours	Improves with time	Irritability, restlessness
Hypertension		Uncontrolled B P

The treatment of stroke consists of prevention of recurrence, prevention of complications and reducing the aftermath of ischemia. Prevention of recurrence of stroke is by the use of Aspirin, the dosage for which is still not fully established, but it varies from 75 mg to 150 mg. It produces irreversible inhibition of platelet function by inactivation of cyclo-oxygenase. Early administration reduces mortality by almost 25 %. Second drug now in use is Ticlopidine in the dosage of 250 mg twice daily. It irreversibly inhibits adenosine diphosphate pathway in platelet metabolism. It also reduces fibrinogen and increases erythrocyte deformability. Recently, Clopidrogel has been introduced, which is administered in the dosage of 75 mg. daily. It is a platelet adenosine diphosphate receptor antagonist. Finally, recent trials have suggested the use of combination of Dypiramidole, 200 mg twice daily with Aspirin in the dose of 25 mg twice daily. It reduces the side effects of Aspirin. Low molecular weight heparin is not recommended for an evolving stroke. In selected cases, unfractionated heparin in the dose of 1000 units per hour may be used intravenously. With non-valvular auricular fibrillation, and anterior wall myocardial infarcts, the use of oral anticoagulent like Warfarin is advocated. The INR should be maintained around 2-3. It is not advised for left ventricular aneurysm and mural thrombi. Intravenous heparin is better for embolism from the carotid artery with stenosis and ulcerated plaques. It should not be used if the infarct size is large or there is presence of haemorrhagic infarct and cerebral oedema.

If the infarct is large and there is rise of intracranial pressure, endotracheal intubation should be carried out and hyperventilation done. Judicious use of Mannitol is advised especially in the elderly where the chances of renal shut down are high. Patient must be maintained euvolimic by measuring pressure on the antibiotic coated central venous line.

Thrombolytic therapy has to be given within three hours from the onset of the symptoms. For thrombolytic therapy by rtPA, the patient should report before 3 hours of stroke, without seizure at the onset, and with normal blood sugar or at least not below 50 mg/dl or above 400 mg/dl. There should be no prior history of haemorrhagic stroke, gastrointestinal bleeding or genito-urinary bleeding. Presence of recent myocardial infarction is also a contraindication. The blood pressure should not be higher than 185/110. There should not be a history of current use of anticoagulants and the platelet count should not be below 100,000. Finally, there should be no history of serious head injury or recent major surgery. CT scan of the brain must exclude cerebral haemorrhage or haemorrhagic infarction. Use of streptokinase for this purpose is now contraindicated. Trials are on for the use of Ancrod, an extract from the venom of Malaysian pit viper.

The value of Nimodipine, a calcium channel blocker has not been established for the management of stroke. It is important that the airways are kept patent to prevent hypoxia and hypercarbia and if need be an endotracheal tube must be inserted. It is equally important to maintain normal temperature and hyperpyrexia avoided. Diabetes and diabetic acidosis should be treated. Sublingual nifedipine or intravenous labotalol is administered if the blood pressure in above180 mm systolic. Cardiac failure should be treated. Patient should not be allowed to become hypovolemic by maintenance of fluid balance. Electrolytes should be checked regularly. Aspiration pneumonia should be prevented by correct posture and if need be intragastric tube. Myocardial ischemia coexists in 3 per cent of cases and should be attended to simultaneously. Finally due nursing care be given for prevention of bedsores etc.

It is now established that if the carotid artery stenosis with parenchymal events, exceeds 70 per cent of the original lumen of the artery, stenting or endarterectomy should be carried out. Surgery is also suggested in asymptomatic carotid artery stenosis. Surgical risk, morbidity and mortality increase in the inexperienced hands. Conversion to a haemorrhagic stroke is the most likely complication, despite this surgery or stenting is recommended. It is also safe to consider endarterectomy for critical stenosis of the carotid artery after thrombolytic therapy for thrombosis of the middle cerebral artery.

VENOUS THROMBOSIS is common in India and forms 4.5 % of all obstretic admissions in the hospital. Of all cases of venous thrombosis 60 % are due to puerperal sepsis, dehydration and CCF forms another 15 % and pyogenic and TB meningitis another 15 %. The remaining 10 % are due to large number of factors listed below. It is met with in 15-30 % of post-partum state due either to regional sepsis, injury or surgery. The other causes for venous thrombosis in women are the use of contraceptive pills containing oestrogen or hyper-coagulable state during pregnancy. There are many other factors responsible for venous thrombosis, such as use of androgens for body building, cyanotic heart disease or congestive cardiac failure, deficiency of antithrombin III, protein S and C, homocysteinemia, antiphospholipid syndrome with labile hypertension and recurrent abortions, use of cancer chemotherapy, leukaemia, polycythemia, dehydration and nephrotic syndrome.

The superficial cerebral veins drain into cavernous sinus, the thrombosis of which is due to spread of infection from face. Patient presents with fever, chills, and toxaemia. There is proptosis, chemosis and ophthalmoplegia, unilateral initially later bilateral. Papilloedema and haemorrhages in the retina indicate retinal vein thrombosis. Optic nerve is usually normal. Fungal infection due to uncontrolled diabetes is common. The inferior cerebral vein drains into lateral sinus. The vein of Galen drains the thalamus and the basal ganglia into the inferior sagittal sinus. Thrombosis of vein of Galen produces hydrocephalus, and infarcts in thalamus and basal ganglia. The superior sagittal sinus and the basal system of veins are well connected through the veins of Labbe and Trolard. Thrombosis of the superior sagittal sinus or lateral sinus produces rise in intracranial pressure and focal fits. Cortical paraplegia or crural monoplegia, with cortical sensory loss in the legs and bladder symptoms form the classical picture of superior sagittal sinus thrombosis. Due to thrombosis of the cortical veins, the brain is swollen, with oedema. There is mottled grey cyanotic discoloration of the surface of the brain with blood stained meninges. The thrombosis of the veins on the superior surface leads to a haemorrhagic infarct. The central part resembles a haematoma, surrounded by softened brain. Patient presents with multifocal seizures, fleeting neurological deficit such as aphasia, apraxia, and cortical blindness and declining sensorium during the second week. Bilateral papilloedema is noted with signs of raised intracranial pressure. If compression of the Jugular vein on one side produces swelling of the veins of face, scalp and retina, it suggests thrombosis of jugular vein or transverse sinus on the opposite side. Similarly, the CSF pressure fails to rise after jugular compression because of the thrombosis of lateral sinus. The treatment consists of antiepileptic agents if convulsions are present. Use of unfractionated heparin is indicated if there is no parenchymal haemorrhage. In the presence of haemorrhage, it may have to be used very carefully. The role of low molecular heparins is unclear at this point in time. Rarely, direct injection of thrombolytic agents has been successfully performed. The intracranial pressure may rise due to the blockage of the venous outflow and will need to be treated with cerebral decongestants like mannitol and glycerol. The cause of the venous sinus thrombosis will also need attention. Prognosis is good in idiopathic cases and in symptomatic cases; the underlying condition decides the outcome.

CEREBRAL HAEMORRHAGE: Cerebral haemorrhage can result from many different causes.

Table 7.4

Causes Of Cerebral Haemorrhage

Causes
Hypertension
Arterio-venous malformation
Bleeding diathesis
Mycotic aneurysm
Arteritis
Haemorrhagic leukoencephalopathy
Head injury
Aneurysm
Anticoagulation
Haemorrhage in tumour, cyst, abscess
Amyloid angiopathy
Idiopathic

The commonest cause of cerebral haemorrhage is rupture of a micro aneurysm in a patient with history of hypertension. It is more common in males than females. It occurs commonly after the age of 60 years. The internal capsule is the commonest site of haemorrhage. The next common sites are thalamus and basal ganglia. The thalamic haemorrhage can bleed into the ventricles. The other sites are various lobes, cerebellum and pons. Parietal and frontal haemorrhages are more frequent than temporal and occipital. With massive haemorrhage, coma develops rapidly, the pulse rate is slow and the breathing is stertorous. 'Cheyne-Stokes' respiration may occur. The head and eyes look at the lesion. If blood has seeped into the subarachnoid space, the patient may be markedly restless. He may move the unaffected side continuously. The hemiplegia is initially flaccid. The diagnosis is easily made by a CAT scan examination. Around the area of haemorrhage, there may be areas of ischemia and oedema. The mortality rises with the size of haemorrhage and oedema.

The pontine haemorrhage results in facial paralysis on the side of the lesion and hemiplegia on the contralateral side. The eyes look to the opposite side due to paralysis of the conjugate gaze on the side of the lesion. Initially the signs may be unilateral but as the haemorrhage extends the signs become bilateral and extensive. The patient is comatose, with pinpoint pupils, bilateral facial weakness, and loss of eye movements. However, the eyes may move on Doll's eye manoeuvre. There is quadriplegia with bilateral extensor plantar responses. No gag reflex is elicited and there is inability to swallow. Haemorrhages generally develop during the day when the patient is active. Loss of consciousness occurs early in the course of the disease. Blood in the CSF suggests extension into the subarachnoid space or ventricles.

TREATMENT consists of general measures. The blood pressure if very high should be lowered. Hyperthermia and hypovolemia should be prevented. Oxygenation should be maintained with endotracheal tube and thus aspiration pneumonia prevented. General measures as outlined for management of stroke earlier need to be carried out. If there is rise in intracranial pressure, corticosteroids and mannitol should be used. Surgery is indicated for massive lobar bleeds but usually not for thalamic or deeper haemorrhages.

Primary subarachnoid haemorrhage due to rupture of an aneurysm or arterio-venous malformation is differentiated from intracerebral haemorrhage by the initial symptoms. There is a sudden onset of severe unrelenting headache. Vomiting may also occur. Signs of meningeal irritation such as neck stiffness, Kernig's sign and Brudzinski's sign are present. If the bleed is severe or it has burst into the cerebral substance, various stages of coma may develop with focal neurological signs. Aneurysms are more common in the anterior circulation. They need to be diagnosed by scanning – CT or MRI, MR angiography and later digital subtraction angiography. They need to be attended to early, to prevent recurrent bleed, which is almost always fatal. Small aneurysms of the size of 2-3 mm rarely bleed and may be left untreated. The patient must have a yearly angiogram to verify the size and growth. Introduction of coils or surgical clamping, depending on the site and size of the aneurysm is the line of treatment.

CHAPTER VIII

NEUROMUSCULAR DISORDERS

CLINICAL APPROACH: When faced with a patient with the problem of weakness of muscles, the initial clinical step is to differentiate between the upper motor neuron and the lower motor neuron lesions. This differentiation is usually not difficult, based on the distribution of the weakness and the associated symptoms and signs as discussed earlier. When analysing the lower motor neuron diseases, following five anatomical levels of affectation need to be considered.

1. Anterior horn cells
2. Roots
3. Peripheral nerves
4. Neuromuscular junction
5. Muscles

The distribution of weakness, symmetry and presence of sensory symptoms and signs can help the clinician to derive the site of the disease process.

Diseases of the neuromuscular junction, for example myasthenia gravis and the various other congenital myasthenic syndromes have a very suggestive symptomatology. They have preferential affection of the eye movements and the pharyngeal musculature resulting in diplopia and dysphagia. Fatigue and diurnal variation are characteristic and help in the diagnosis. Fatigue should be differentiated from weakness. The first contraction is normal in fatigue and the strength progressively decreases with successive contractions. In other diseases producing weakness, even the first effort will be suboptimal.

Besides the fatigue and fluctuating weakness of the preferred areas, myasthenic patients do not have any change in the muscle bulk, tone and the deep tendon reflexes, thus making it easy for the clinician to spot them. Occasionally, the symptoms manifest only in the limbs and this may need very careful assessment.

Radiculopathies have pain as the clinical hallmark and result in asymmetrical, painful, proximal and distal sensory and motor syndrome. Disc disease, tuberculosis, viral and spirochetal infections are some of the common causes of radiculopathies.

Unlike radiculopathy, distal and symmetrical sensori-motor deficits are likely to be caused by peripheral neuropathies. Peripheral neuropathies result either due to axonal degeneration (axonopathies) or due to myelin disorders (myelinopathies). The distal and symmetrical nature is seen more consistently with axonopathies. Axonopathies usually result from toxic or metabolic causes and follow the principle of length dependency. The length dependency principle states that longer axons will suffer first as it is difficult for the cell body to provide nourishment to the tips of the longer axons and also to clear the waste products and toxins from them. Hence the axonopathic peripheral neuropathies begin distally and symmetrically in soles and progress upwards. By the time the symptoms reach the mid shin area, the complaints begin in upper extremities, initially in the fingers and then the symptoms proceed centripetally. Demyelination of the peripheral nervous system, on the other hand, being focal and segmental by its very nature, need not follow the above-mentioned principle. In practice, we see patients with Guillain-Barre syndrome begin with weakness of the thighs before the feet or begin with the cranial nerves and descend to the longer limb nerves. Another point of note is that acquired neuropathies produce more symptoms than signs (e.g. diabetic neuropathy) where as asymptomatic patients having very slowly progressive hereditary neuropathies can have devastating sensory deficits. This point has exceptions e.g. Hansen's disease.

Loss of deep tendon reflexes is most consistently seen in patients with sensori-motor peripheral neuropathies and the dictum that there is no peripheral neuropathy without ankle areflexia is usually true. Exceptions are small fibre neuropathies like diabetes mellitus, hereditary sensory autonomic neuropathy, Fabry's disease etc. but besides diabetes, other small fibre neuropathies are rare in clinical practice. Neuropathies generally result in mixed sensori-motor deficits but one component may be dominant.

Table 8.1

Motor or Sensory Neuropathies

MAINLY MOTOR NEUROPATHIES	MAINLY SENSORY NEUROPATHIES
Hereditary sensory motor Neuropathy	Hereditary autonomic sensory neuropathy
Guillain-Barre syndrome	Diabetes
Lead toxicity	Systemic lupus erythematosus
Acute motor axonal neuropathy	Amyloidosis
Multifocal motor neuropathy	Fabry's disease
Osteosclerotic myeloma	Tangier's disease
Porphyria	

The table below lists the causes of peripheral neuritis:

Table 8.2

Etiological classification of neuropathies

I. Acquired

A. Metabolic

1. Diabetes (Polyneuropathgy, autonomic neuropathies, mononeuropathies, cranial neuropathies)
2. Uremia
3. Hypothyroidism (esp. carpal tunnel syndrome)
4. Acromegaly
5. Addison's disease
6. Liver failure

B. Nutritional

1. Mixed (alcoholism, malnutrition, dietary fads, malabsorption syndrome)
2. Beriberi
3. Pellagra
4. B12 deficiency
5. B6 deficiency

C. Toxins.

1. Heavy metals (lead, mercury, gold, arsenic, thallium)

2. Drugs (Vincristine, INH, Dapsone, Nitrofurantoin, Disulfiram, Perhexilene, Hydralazine, Amiodarone)
3. Organo-phosphate compounds (Tri-o-cresyl phosphate)
4. Acrylamide
5. Volatile hydrocarbons (n-hexane, methyl-n-butyl ketone)
6. Cobra venom

D. Infections

1. Leprosy
2. Diphtheria
3. Herpes zoster
4. Botulism

E. Presumed Immunologic

1. Serum sickness (esp. Brachial plexus)
2. Inflammatory
    a. Motor polyradiculoneuropathy (Guillain-Barre syndrome)
    b. Sensory polyradiculoneuropathy
    c. Autonomic neuropathy
    d. Cranial polyneuropathy

F. Collagen-vascular

1. Polyarteritis Nodosa
2. Rheumatoid arthritis
3. Systemic Lupus Erythematosus
4. Scleroderma
5. Dermatomyositis-polymyositis

G. Ischemic vascular disease

H. Remote effects of cancer

1. Multiple myeloma and other dysproteinemias
2. Carcinomatous neuromyopathy

I. Trauma and compression (entrapment neuropathies of both upper lower limbs)

J. Tumours

1. Primary (Neurinomas, neurofibromas)
2. Secondary

K. Miscellaneous

1. Sarcoidosis

2. Primary Amyloidosis

II. Genetically determined neuropathies

A. Hereditory motor sensory neuropathy (HMSN)

1. Charcot-Marie-Tooth disease
2. Dejerine-Sottas disease
3. Refsum's disease

B. Hereditary sensory neuropathy

1. Neuropathy of Denny-Brown
2. Riley-Dey syndrome
3. Familial dysautonomia
4. Congenital insensitivity to pain

C. Heredofamilial amyloidosis

D. Leuckodystrophies

1. Metachromatic lekodystrophy
2. Fabry's disease (Diffuse angiokeratosis)
3. Krabbe's globoid cell leukodystrophy

E. Others

1. Acute intermittent porphyria
2. Bassen-Kornweiz disease (Abetalipoproteinemia)
3. Tangier's disease (A-alphalipoproteinemia)

Neuropathies may also have severe pain and dysasthesiae as the presenting and the dominant feature and this helps the differential diagnosis.

Table 8.3

Painful Neuropathies

Diabetes mellitus	Vasculitis
Thiamine deficiency	Pyridoxine deficiency
Paraneoplastic neuropathy	Amyloidosis
Uraemia	Arsenic poisoning
Thallium toxicity	Vincristine use
INH	Fabry's disease
Alcohol abuse	HIV infection

Neuropathies like Guillain-Barre syndrome, diabetes, porphyria and amyloidosis may have significant autonomic involvement. At times, polyneuropathies may be associated with optic nerve dysfunction.

Table 8.4

Polyneuropathies With Visual Impairment

Vitamin B 12 deficiency
Thallium poisoning
Systemic lupus erythematosus
Diabetes mellitus
Subacute myelo-optic neuropathy
Strachan syndrome
Dapsone use
Disulfiram use
Refsum's disease
Tobacco alcohol amblyopia and neuropathy

The most challenging clinical problem arises when trying to decide whether a pure motor disorder is due to anterior horn cell disease or to a muscle disease. Following points help the differentiation.

Table 8.5

Differentiation between Anterior Horn Cell Diseases and Myopathies

Anterior horn cell disease	Myopathies
Asymmetric	Symmetrical
Distal and proximal	Usually proximal
Mild or no hypertropy	Marked hypertropy may be present
Wasting more than weakness	Weakness more than wasting
Fasciculations seen	Almost never
Eelectrophysiology shows Giant units, increased insertional activity and fallout of motor units	Small amplitude short duration polyphasic potentials, normal insertional activity and full or overfull recruitment

Deep tendon reflexes have purposely been left out of this table. The areflexia seems to be most tightly linked to the sensori-motor affectations like peripheral neuropathies and the radiculopathies. However, areflexia is less helpful in differentiation of pure motor conditions. There is a general observation that the deep tendon reflexes tend to be sluggish or absent earlier in the course of anterior horn cell diseases as compared to myopathies. However, patients with Duchenne muscular dystrophy regularly loose the knee reflex at a stage when the quadriceps is mildly weak and the child is walking Pronounced muscle hypertrophy is mainly seen in myogenic diseases. Neurogenic conditions may have mild hypertrophy. Table 8.6 lists the causes of calf hypertrophy.

DISORDERS OF MUSCLE:

Myopathy is a broad term, which encompasses all diseases of muscle. Muscle diseases may be divided in to hereditary and acquired. Hereditary conditions are

1. Muscular dystrophies
2. Myotonias
3. Periodic paralysis
4. Storage disorders
5. Mitochondrial cytopathies
6. Congenital myopathies

MUSCULAR DYSTROPHIES: The term dystrophy means an inherited, progressive, primary disease of muscle with degeneration and regeneration of muscle fibres. In view of their inherited nature, muscular dystrophies are best classified according to the mode of inheritance.

X-LINKED MUSCULAR DYSTROPHIES:

This group comprises of Duchenne muscular dystrophy, Becker muscular dystrophy and Emery-Dreifuss muscular dystrophy.

DUCHENNE MUSCULAR DYSTROPHY (DMD): DMD is the commonest muscular dystrophy of childhood with worldwide distribution and an incidence of about 1 in 4000 live male births. Being an X-linked disease, boys are affected. Girls suffer rarely, when they have Turner's syndrome, mosaicism or an X and autosomal translocation. Affected boys are normal at birth but begin showing symptoms at 4-5 years of age. They tend to fall on uneven surfaces and have difficulty in rising. They get up by using Gower's manoeuvre in which they steady the hands on the legs and gradually rise up. They have difficulty in climbing the staircases. The calf muscles at this stage are hypertropied. They have a waddling gait. Weakness of hip flexors results in inability to clear the ground hence; titting the body to opposite side raises the peivis on the side of the advancing foot. This side-to-side movement to advance forwards is known as waddling.

Table 8.6

Causes Of Calf Hypertrophy
Duchenne muscular dystrophy
Becker muscular dystrophy
Hypohyroidism
Cystcercosis, trichinosis
Sarcoglycanopathies, other muscular dystrophies and spinal muscular atrophies

DMD is a disease where the calf hypertrophy is very prominent. The examination, in addition to calf hypertrophy shows weakness of pelvic girdle, trunk and shoulder girdle muscles. The weakness advances rapidly and tendo-achilles contracture develops, resulting in toe walking. This is one of the most severe dystrophy and by the age of 10 years, the children are bound to the wheel chair. At this stage, the spinal muscle weakness results in scoliosis and respiratory difficulties. Cardiac muscle is also affected in two third of the patients and some times is severe enough to manifest clinically with dilated cardiomyopathy. Approximately 70% of such children affected by DMD are of subnormal intelligence, which does not get much worse with the advancement of the muscle disease.

Serum CK is very much elevated, usually in thousands of units (100 or 1000 times the normal), in the early part of the disease and decreases, as the muscles get more and more weak. Electrocardiogram shows right ventricular strain pattern with intermittent bundle branch block and echocardiogram may show evidence of cardiomyopathy.

Table 8.7:

Myopathies With Cardiac Involvement

Duchenne and Becker muscular dystrophy
Myotonic muscular dystrophy
Emery-Dreifuss muscular dystrophy
Mitochondrial disorders
Limb girdle muscular dystrophy IB
Desminopathy
Debrancher enzyme deficiency
Polymyositis

Electromyography shows findings of primary muscle disease and muscle biopsy confirms changes of dystrophy.

Till 1986, not much was known about the molecular events taking place in this disease. Rather fortunately, at this time, a female patient showing features of DMD was studied genetically. She had an X autosome translocation and helped to focus on the translocated short arm of the X chromosome. This portion was soon decoded and the gene was identified at the Xp21site. At this stage, the product of this gene was not known. Rapidly, the DMD gene was fully sequenced. This is one of largest human genes having 79 exons and almost 2000 base pairs. The gene codes for a protein of 428 Kd, the Dystrophin, which is located sub-sarcolemmally and is believed to be a part of the cytoskeleton.

Currently it has become possible to study the deletions in this gene and to estimate the amount of Dystrophin on the fresh frozen muscle. These advances are of enormous significance as they have increased diagnostic accuracy and more importantly, have brought prenatal diagnosis, carrier detection and prevention, to a reality.

BECKER MUSCULAR DYSTROPHY (BMD):

This muscular dystrophy clinically is like a slower version of DMD. Affected males start becoming weak by the age of 8-10 years and the progression is much slower. Cardiac involvement and mental subnormality is less common and the pattern of muscular weakness is the same.

BMD is genetically similar to DMD, with the defect being at the same site of Xp 21. However, the defect is of such a nature that the remaining gene fragment can result in an abbreviated dystrophin, which can retain some function. The genetic testing and counselling is similar to DMD.

AUTOSOMAL RECESSIVE AND AUTOSOMAL DOMINANT MUSCULAR DYSTROPHIES:

These muscular dystrophies are grouped under the broad heading of limb girdle muscular dystrophies. At least 15 well-delineated entities are included under this heading, and there are others that await modern inputs.

As a group, these muscular dystrophies begin in the second and third decade of life and are slowly progressive in their course. Hip girdle is usually affected earlier, producing difficulty in getting up from squatting position followed by the weakness of muscles of trunk and upper girdle. Depending upon the case in consideration, a differential weakness may be detected in the clinical examination. Serum CK is mildly elevated and electromyography reveals myogenic features. The routine muscle biopsy shows changes of muscular dystrophy and oligoclonal antibodies used on the fresh frozen muscle, show specific muscle protein abnormalities.

In the past few years, like in the cases of DMD and BMD, there have been long strides in the elucidation of the genetic and immunocytochemical information in this group of muscular dystrophies and accurate diagnosis, counselling and prevention is now possible in some of these devastating conditions. Sarcoglycans are the proteins mainly involved in this kind of dystrophy. Some of the other proteins, which may be affected, are Dysferlin and Calpain.

CONGENITAL MYOPATHIES: This is an uncommon group of myopathies, as compared to muscular dystrophies. Here, the muscle fibres have defects during early maturation. In this respect, they are very different from muscular dystrophies where in the muscle fibres initially mature normally and then undergo degeneration and regeneration.

In keeping with the fact that the fibres do not mature in early life, these myopathies present themselves at or very soon after birth. The affected children are floppy, i.e. have loose and flabby muscles and have delay in achieving motor milestones. However, it must be remembered that these defective muscle fibres do not usually undergo further changes, or do so minimally. Hence, the children gradually improve in their motor function. On clinical examination, they have very thin muscles (only skin and bones) but on testing the strength is usually better than the appearance of the muscles.

There are few clinical markers to suggest the type of congenital myopathy e.g. the thin and long faces and high arched palate in cases of Nemaline myopathy and ptosis and external ophthalmoplegia in cases of central core disease. However, the type of congenital myopathy is decided largely by studying the muscle biopsy. The biopsy has to be studied for histology and electron microscopy. Following types of congenital myopathies may be defined by the biopsy changes.

1. Nemaline myopathy
2. Central core disease
3. Mini-core and multi-core disease
4. Fibre type disproportion
5. Myopathies with para crystalline inclusions
6. Finger body myopathy etc.

MYOTONIC DISORDERS: This group of conditions is characterized by myotonia. Myotonia is the inability to relax a contracted muscle. Myotonia can be elicited clinically by asking the patient to grip firmly for 15 to 30 seconds and then release the grip. Patients having myotonia will have difficulty in relaxing the handgrip (grip myotonia). Percussion can also elicit it with the hammer; where in the contracted part of muscle stands out as a lump for a while, before subsiding (percussion myotonia).

MYOTONIAS:

1. Myotonic dystrophy
2. Myotonia congenita
3. Paramyotonia
4. Chondrodystrophic myotonia

Myotonic dystrophy is an autosomal dominant disease and is related to increased number of CTG repeats in the tissues. The disease has multi-system involvement and besides the striated muscle, it involves other systems producing cataracts, baldness, mental subnormality and reproductive difficulties. Amongst the striated muscles, it preferentially affects the facial muscles, sternomastoids and distal muscles of the limbs. This pattern of involvement is rather uncommon in myopathies.

Table 8.8:

Myopathies With Facial Weakness

Fascio-scapulo-humeral muscular dystrophy
Myotonic muscular dystrophy
Oculo-pharyngeal muscular dystrophy
Mitochondrial disorders
Congenital myopathies: central core, nemaline, centronuclear
Myasthenia gravis
Myasthenic syndromes

Maternal transmission usually results in more severe disease and the newborn child may present with floppiness. The myotonia responds to membrane stabilizers like Phenytoin, but the weakness does not. Other manifestations of the disease need to be treated symptomatically.

MYOTONIA CONGENITA: Myotonia congenita can be autosomal recessive or dominant disease. Here, unlike the myotonic dystrophy, there are no extramuscular manifestations. The main feature is myotonia and the patients often have out standing muscular development and get a Herculean appearance. Weakness is late and minimal. Since the myotonia is the main feature, response to membrane stabilizers like Phenytoin and Carbamazepine is usually satisfactory.

PERIODIC PARALYSIS: These diseases result from alteration in the concentration of potassiumions in the muscle cells. Depending upon the level of serum potassium, they are divided in to

1. Hypokalmic periodic paralysis
2. Hyperkalemic periodic paralysis
3. Normokalemic periodic paralysis

The clinical features are of episodic weakness of large limb muscles without changes in the deep tendon reflexes. The respiratory muscles are usually not affected. Differences in the three forms of periodic paralyses are outlined below.

Table 8.9

Differences Between Hyper And Hypo Kalemic Periodic Paralysis

	Hyperkalemic	**Paramyotonia congenita**	**Hypokalemic**
Inheritance	Autosomal dominant	Autosomal dominant	Autosomal dominant
Gene	17q	-	1q31.32
Channel	Sodium	Sodium	Calcium
Age of onset	First few weeks of school	Early childhood	2nd Decade
Sex	Both	Both	Males predominant
Provocative factors	Exposure to K Exposure to cold Rest after exercise	Exposure to cold Steady contraction	Heavy carbohydrate meal, Heavy exercise – sleep onset in morning Exposure to steroids, epinephrine
Paralysis	Moderate	Mild	Severe.
Laboratory	High CK & K	–	Low K
EMG	Fibrillations & myotonia on cooling	Myotonic discharges	Not characteristic
ECG	Changes hyperkalemia	– –	Bradycardia, prolonged PR & QT intervals, Flat T, prominent 'U'
Muscle Biopsy	Tubular aggregates & vacuoles	Variation of fibre size, occ.vacuole	Myopathic changes, vacuoles, tubular aggregates
Treatment	Sugar candy sweet drinks, IV calcium, NaCl,	Avoid cold	Fruit juices, oral K Low Na, carbohydrate diet
Prevention	Acetazolamide, dichlorophenamide		Acetazolamide, Dichlorophenamide

STORAGE DISORDERS: This group of disorders results due to inherited abnormalities of metabolic enzymes required in the catabolism of substrates like glycogen, lipids etc. These diseases present in childhood with exercise intolerance. As the patient exercises, cramps and weakness develops in the exercised muscles. At times myoglobinuria can occur. Rest restores strength. In lipid storage disorders, after the initial exercise induced symptoms; the patient may be able to continue muscular activity for some more time. This is labelled as the second wind phenomenon.

Depending on the type of enzymatic deficiency, the symptoms vary. Diagnosis is made on histology of the muscle, which shows inclusions containing glycogen or lipids. No curative therapy is available but explanation of precipitating factors and conservative measures during the episodes is usually successful in maintaining active lifestyle in most patients. If the myonecrosis is very severe during an acute episode, renal insufficiency due to blockage of tubules by myoglobin may develop, requiring dialysis.

MITOCHONDRIAL CYTOPATHIES: These disorders are comparatively newly recognized. They are transmitted maternally as sperm has few or no mitochondria. Mitochondria are universal in distribution and hence there are many organs involved in these diseases. Muscle is one of the preferentially affected organs. Weakness is the chief manifestation and ocular movements are more commonly involved. The key to the diagnosis is multi-organ involvement. A wide variety of clinical presentations are known. The well-recognized patterns are the Kearns-Syres syndrome (short stature, external ophthalmoplegia, heart blocks etc), MELAS (myoclonic epilepsy, lactic acidosis and stroke like episodes) and the MERRF (myoclonus, encephalopathy and ragged red fibbers). Estimating lactate and pyruvate levels in serum helps to arrive at the diagnosis. Diagnosis is further substantiated by demonstration of accumulation of abnormal mitochondria in the muscle fibre, by special stains like the Gomori trichrome stain. Further, specific biochemical enzymatic deficiency may be estimated by tissue analysis and therapy can be directed to providing the cofactor helpful in the defective enzymatic reactions.

POLYMYOSITIS AND DERMATOMYOSITIS:

The muscle may be inflamed due to a variety of infections. Viruses like Coxsackie B, Echo, adenovirus, herpes simplex, Epstein Barr virus and mycoplasma can produce myositis. Trichinosis, toxoplasmosis, and other protozoan and fungal infections can affect the muscles. Sarcoidosis produces non-caseating granulomata in the muscles.

When idiopathic inflammation of the striated muscles is encountered, the term polymyositis is used. Dermatomyositis refers to additional involvement of the skin. Polymyositis presents with subacute weakness of the proximal limb muscles, which is insidious and progressive. Muscle ache may be present. The swallowing may also be affected in some patients. Cardiac arrhythmias and decreased efficiency of the myocardial pump is also known. In cases of dermatomyositis, there are skin lesions preferentially seen around the eyelids, on the knuckles and the chest region. In Indian people, the colour of he skin rashes is red brown. Both, polymyositis and dermatomyositis are associated with connective tissue disorders and carcinomas. They may precede the development of the malignancy by few months. Laboratory tests reveal very high levels of muscle enzymes, usually the CPK values are in thousands. Additionally, laboratory tests may detect collagenosis or show the presence of malignancy. Electrophysiology shows evidence of myopathy and the spontaneous activity may be increased. The muscle biopsy confirms presence of interstitial inflammatory exudate and shows degenerating and regenerating muscle fibres. In cases of dermatomyositis, the blood vessels may show presence of inflammation in their walls. Such patients tend to have perifascicular muscle fibre atrophy, due to ischaemia.

Treatment is initially begun with corticosteroids, 1 mg/kg body weight and the patient monitored clinically and with CPK levels. Steroids are gradually tapered. In some patients it is possible to stop them totally, in others, a small maintenance dose is needed and some others may require addition of another immunosuppressant like the Azathioprine or Methotrexate. Prognosis is usually satisfactory. When the inflammatory myopathy is a part of the systemic disease, the prognosis depends upon the underlying condition.

DRUG RELATED MYOPATHIES

A wide variety of drugs are capable of producing myopahties and the syndromes are often related to the duration and the dosage of the offending agent. It is therefore important to inquire the details of drug intake when dealing with a patient of myopathy.

Table 8.10

Drug Related Myopathies

Types of Myopathies	Drugs
Rhabdomyolysis	Alcohol, Heroin, Barbiturates, Epsilon aminocaproic acid
Acute/subacute painful necrotising myopathy	Clofibrate, Vincristine, Emetine
Hypokalemic myopathy	Diuretics, Amphotericin B
Inflammatory myopathy	D-penicillamine, Procainamide,
Subacute/chronic painless myopathy	Corticosteroids, Chloroquine
Focal myonecrosis	Chlorpromazine, Antibiotics

DISEASES OF THE PERIPHERAL NERVES:

Peripheral nerve diseases are grouped as

1. Mononeuropathies
2. Mononeuritis multiplex
3. Polyneuropathies

MONONEUROPATHIES: The term means affectation of a single nerve. Single nerve affectations are usually seen at pressure points and at entrapment sites, for example, ulnar nerve affectation at elbow, lateral popliteal nerve at fibula, median nerve at carpal tunnel etc. The aetiologies of mononeuropathies are Hansen's disease, diabetes, compressions and entrapments. The treatment depends upon the cause of the mononeuropathy. Entrapments require appropriate surgical decompressions and specific primary medical conditions need medical therapy.

Table 8.11

Common Entrapment Syndromes

Nerve	Site of Compression
Suprascapular nerve	Spinoglenoid notch
Radial nerve	Humeral groove
Median nerve	Carpel tunnel
Ulnar nerve	Cubital tunnel
Ulnar nerve	Palmar fascia-pisiform bone
Anterior interosseous nerve	Between 2 heads of pronator muscle
Lateral cutaneous nerve of thigh	Inguinal ligament
Obturator nerve	Obturator canal
Lateral poplitial nerve	Head of fibula
Posterior tibial nerve	Tarsal tunnel

MONONEURITIS MULTIPLEX (MM): The term MM implies affectation of multiple nerves. This results in an asymmetrical process of peripheral neuropathy. When dealing with such patients, the initial part of history is important. The patient should be asked how and where the disease began and the chronological order of the symptoms. Often the disease affects initially one digit, followed by other digits. This is very important to elucidate, as advancing MM will ultimately turn in to a polyneuropathy when many nerves are affected. In patients with MM, dysaesthesiae are a prominent feature, which perhaps makes the patients present early to the doctor.

The causes of MM are:

1. Hansen's disease
2. Collagen vascular diseases like polyarteritis nodosa, rheumatoid arthritis, SLE, Wagener's granulomatosis etc.
3. Diabetes mellitus
4. MM presentation of CIDP
5. Sarcoidosis
6. Carcinomas
7. Paraproteinemias and cryoglobulinemia
8. Intravenous drug use and abuse

ESR, ANA, DsDNA, HBsAg, blood sugar level and electrophysiology are helpful. Electromyography and nerve conduction study is particularly important as it has the ability to confirm MM even when the clinical presentation has become symmetrical. It is important to recognize MM as definitive therapy is available and the results are rewarding. Besides treating the primary condition, in immune mediated MM, corticosteroids and immunoglobulins are useful.

POLYNEUROPATHIES: Polyneuropathies are either axonopathies or myelinopathies, Axonopathies are often related to deficiency states, toxins, and metabolic and endocrine abnormalities. They present as length dependant distal symmetrical sensori-motor deficits.

Myelinopathies can be hereditary or acquired. Hereditary myelinopathies are exemplified by the Charcot-Marie-Tooth disease or gradually progressive hereditary motor sensory neuropathy, Acquired myelinopathies are immune mediated and hence are focal and segmental by nature. Hence they may not follow the length dependency principle.

GUILLAIN-BARRE SYNDROME (GBS): GBS is an acute inflammatory demyelinating polyradiculoneuropathy. It affects all ages and both sexes. The disease is designated after Guillain- Barre, Landry and Strohl. Landry initially described it in 1859 and the others wrote about it in 1916. GBS forms one of the common causes of rapidly progressive weakness. GBS has increasingly become important in clinical neurology, as it is rapidly diagnosable and potentially treatable. The disease can affect respiratory, bulbar and autonomic functions and often requires critical neurological and medical care.

ANTECEDENT EVENTS: Two third of patients have history of infectious illness 2-4 weeks prior to the neurological symptoms. Flu like illness or diarrhoea due to a variety of agents including Campylobactor jejuni is common but Mycoplasma, Chlamydia, Borrelia and HIV may also be encountered. Vaccinations, surgery and conditions altering immunity like the collagen vascular diseases and lymphoproliferative disorders are other uncommon associations of GBS.

CLINICAL FEATURES: The onset of symptoms is usually subacute and the evolution occurs over 2-3 weeks. Rarely, the symptoms may continue to worsen for up to four weeks. Muscular weakness is the dominant symptom and can affect the proximal and or distal muscles. Weakness is usually symmetrical. Cranial nerves are affected frequently and uni or bi facial involvement is perhaps most frequent. Mild sensory symptoms, pain and paraesthesiae in calves and legs usually accompany the weakness. Deep tendon reflexes are abolished in affected areas soon after the weakness sets in. Of particular importance are bulbar and respiratory functions as their affectation has bearing on the management. Autonomic functions are often abnormal with sympathetic or parasympathetic overactivity resulting in tachycardia and fluctuating hypertension. At times, serious cardiac arrhythmias and arrest can occur.

Table 8.12

Differential Diagnosis of GB Syndrome

DIAGNOSIS	DIFFERENTIATING FEATURES
1. Poliomyelitis	young age, asymmetry, CSF pleocytosis
2. periodic paralysis	repeated attacks, reflexes spared, S. potassium altered
3. Myasthenia gravis	ocular and pharyngeal weakness, reflexes normal, fatiguability
4. Acute intermittent porphyria	coca -cola coloured urine, abdominal pain, h/o drug ingestion, cerebral symptoms/
5. Toxic neuropathy	h/o exposure, skin and hair changes, heavy metal detected in hair and skin
6. Botulinism	prominence of cranial and external ocular weakness, unreactive pupils
7. Diptheritic neuropathy	Young age, pharyngitis early palatal weakness

VARIENT CLINICAL PRESENTATIONS:

1. Pure sensory neuropathy
2. Pure autonomic neuropathy
3. Miller-Fisher syndrome of ataxia, areflexia and opthalmoplegia
4. Axonal type

PATHOGENESIS: GBS is thought to be the result of immune mediated demyelination of the peripheral nervous system. The Schwann cells and myelin are targeted by the immune response, which has both humoral, and cell mediated components. The antigen has not yet been extracted but it is likely to be an infectious agent.

PATHOLOGY: As majority of patients with GBS improve, pathology is not easy to obtain. In the few patients dying of GBS, mononuclear cell infiltration of the endoneurium has been noted. The inflammation affects the whole length from root up to distal nerve twigs but the proximal lesions tend to be more severe. The principle process is of demyelination, though some cases may show axonal degeneration also. Rarely, axonal degeneration may be the main process.

LABORATORY FEATURES: The most consistent abnormalities are seen in the CSF examination and the nerve conduction studies. The CSF examination is usually normal in the first 48-72 hours but by 7-10 days, the protein content is elevated in most of these patients. Hence, 7-10 days is the most appropriate time to perform the CSF examination. Typically, the protein content is elevated to 100-200mg % and cellular response is absent, known as the albumino-cytological dissociation. When GBS occurs in relation with HIV or Lyme disease, the cell count may be elevated.

Nerve conduction studies show slowing of less than 70% of normal, mostly over the proximal segments. Distal motor and sensory latencies may be prolonged. When axonal degeneration takes place, the amplitude of the compound muscle action potential may be reduced. In some cases, the pathology may be restricted to the proximal nerve segments and then the distal NCVs will be normal but the F waves are prolonged. Like the CSF, NCV studies also need 4-5 days to reflect the changes and are best done at 5-10 days interval.

Haematological studies are usually normal unless collagen vascular disease or lymphoproliferative diseases are associated with GBS. IgM antibody against the Epstein-Barr virus and cytomegalo virus may be positive. In selected cases, HIV screening may be undertaken. When diarrhoea is the antecedent event, it is worthwhile sending the stool sample for the isolation of Campylobactor jejuni.

PROGNOSTIC FACTORS: Even though majority of patients has full or nearly total recovery, 10-20% may be left with disability.

1. Older subjects may be left behind with motor disability. Factors indicating poor outcome are age > 60 years
2. Rapid onset and progress
3. Need for artificial ventilation
4. Severely reduced distal compound muscle action potential without dispersion indicating axonal degeneration

THERAPY: A patient with GBS needs admission and observation as the condition progresses in the initial period. The main attention has to be on the respiratory and bulbar dysfunction. When swallowing is affected, Ryle's tube feeding is in order. Blood pressure needs monitoring very carefully as autonomic dysfunction can lead to cardiac arrhythmia and labile hypertension.

Respiratory function is of paramount importance. At the bedside, it can be assessed by single breath count and the ability to hold the breath. Tidal volume measurements can also be performed at the bedside using inexpensive gadgets. Airway should be kept patent and intubation is indicated when the tidal volume drops below 160 mm. and ventilatory assistance may be initiated preferably in an elective manner.

Plasmapharesis and or administration of intravenous immunoglobulins are now recommended as the most effective line of treatment. In plasmapharesis 50 cc of serum/kg body weight is exchanged for plasma or albumin in one cycle and each cycle may be repeated daily or an alternate days till five cycles are over. Four to five grams of immunoglobulin per kg of body weight is given for three to four days.

CHRONIC INFLAMMATORY DEMYELINATING NEUROPATHY: (CIDP)

CIDP is like a stretched out GBS. In this condition, the patient's weakness progresses for longer than four weeks and often for months. The clinical examination usually shows sensory as well as motor deficits, unlike the pure motor weakness seen in GBS.

CIDP results from an immune mediated process of the peripheral nerves, where the antigenic challenge is more persistent than the monophasic antigen presentation of the GBS and therefore the clinical presentation is of a longer evolution. Like most other immune mediated neurological disorders, corticosteroids are the mainstay of therapy. Depending upon the tempo of the illness, one could use injections of Methylprednisolone in the dose of 1 gram per day for three to five days and then follow it up with oral Prednisolone 1 mg/kg/day and then taper as the condition stabilizes. When the patient cannot tolerate steroids or for the fear of side effects, other immunosupressants like the Azathioprine and Methotrexate can be added or substituted. The course is unpredictable. One third of the treated patients improve satisfactorily and the steroid therapy can be discontinued. In the other one-third patients, good clinical outcome can be achieved only with continued immunosupression and the remaining one-third of patients deteriorate despite therapy.

TOXIC NEUROPATHIES: Toxins like the heavy metals (lead, mercury, arsenic, and thallium) and organophosphorus compounds when ingested chronically or acutely can lead to peripheral neuropathy. The sources are usually Ayurvedic medications, lead fumes inhaled due to vehicular pollution and fertilizers consumed due to poor hygiene or insecticides consumed for suicidal attempts. The neuropathy is sensori-motor with dysaesthesiae and pain. Lead neuropathy is an exception, as it results in a pure motor neuropathy. There may be desquamation of skin over the palms and soles and hyperkeratosis. Mee's lines may be seen in the nails following chronic exposure to heavy metals. The diagnostic process begins with clinical suspicion and the proof comes with demonstration of elevated heavy metal levels in the serum, nails, hair and bones. Therapy is related to stopping further exposure and in some cases, chelation to remove the heavy metals from the system. As the neuropathy is painful, symptomatic therapy with Amitryptylline, Gabapentin or Carbamazepine is usually necessary.

DRUG INDUCED NEUROPATHIES: A wide variety of drugs can lead to peripheral neuropathy and the list keeps growing as more and more drugs get introduced. Drug related neuropathies tend to be of the axonal type, resulting in distal, symmetrical sensory motor areflexic deficits. The severity of symptoms usually correlates with dose and duration of exposure. The drugs commonly producing neuropathy have been given below.

1. Isoniazide
2. Dapsone
3. Nitrofurantoin
4. Disulfiram
5. Perhexilene
6. Hydralazine
7. Cordarone
8 Antimalignancy drugs.

Uncommonly, the site of affectation may be the dorsal root ganglion instead of the peripheral nerve, resulting in a ganglionopathy. Such patients have severe sensory loss, usually of the position and the vibration sense. In contrast to the severe sensory loss, the motor system tends to be spared as the site of lesion is away from the motor system. Ganglionopathies are seen with antimalignancy agents like Vincristin, Cis Platin, and Daunorubicin etc.

DEFICIENCY NEUROPATHIES: Deficiency of a variety of vitamins and co factors lead to peripheral neuropathies. As a group, they tend to be symmetrical sensory and mildly motor disorders with prominent sensory phenomena. The important amongst these are the following.

DEFICIENCY OF VITAMIN B 12: Vitamin B 12 is important for the synthesis of nucleic acids in all cells, particularly the actively growing cells such as the mucosal and the hemopoetic cells. Its deficiency is seen in India, not infrequently, as the dietary supplementation is often inadequate in vegetarians in low socio-economic strata. Long religious fasts, ileocoecal granulomatous diseases and alcohol dependence are other factors related to the deficiency.

The symptoms of B_{12} deficiency principally involve the peripheral nerves and result in paraesthesiae of soles with gradual evolution of distal symmetrical sensory deficit. The position and vibration sense is maximally affected; resulting in sensory ataxia, which worsens in the dark. As the disease advances, pyramidal signs, higher mental changes and cerebellar dysfunction also evolve. The laboratory investigations may show haematological abnormalities like megalocytosis and anaemia but the haematological and neurological aspects of B_{12} deficiency can exist independent of each other and the blood picture may be entirely normal. Serum B_{12} levels will, however, be reduced. When the B_{12} levels are in the inconclusive range, further laboratory work up with estimation of methyl malonic acid may be undertaken. Electrophysiological tests show axonal neuropathy and somato-sensory evoked potentials (SSEPs) may be delayed, suggestive of posterior column involvement. MRI shows a characteristic appearance of abnormal signals in the tract of Gall and Burdah, which can help the diagnostic process significantly.

Treatment is rewarding and changes can be reversed. The therapy is begun with injections of Cyanocobalamine 1000 micrograms a day for 15 days and then with tapering frequency. Folic acid supplementation is necessary. A search for the cause of the deficiency should be undertaken, but it can become extensive and expensive.

CHAPTER IX

CRANIO-SPINAL INJURIES

Trauma is a major cause of death around the world. In India it is a common cause of death. Head injuries cause both mortality and morbidity. Since there is no registry for head injuries, it is difficult to state as to how many of the head injuries are serious. However, the casualty department of any large general hospital in India will have 80% of all head injuries as mild injuries, 10 % each as moderate and severe injuries.

The cause of head injury depends on the environment of the patient. Majority of head injuries is due to vehicular accident, specially the accidents on two and three wheelers as wearing of helmet is not compulsory in all the states. In urban areas, overcrowding of trains also is an important cause of accidents. In southern rural areas, fall of coconuts on the head is also an important cause. Other causes are assault with lethal weapons and use of iron or wooden rods, axe, clubs or swords. Falls and recreational injuries are other causes. Head injuries can be blunt, penetrating, open or closed. Open injuries cause CSF leak and infection.

Initial impact sets into motion biochemical and structural changes. Hypoxia, hypovolemia, hypothermia and hypoglycaemia cause further insult, which leads to post-traumatic event, such as raised intra-cranial pressure. When the injury is blunt, delayed axonal injury occurs. The axonal damage is usually in the white matter of cerebrum but when the injury is more severe, it may be combined with either callosal lesion or lesion of the brain stem. The axonal damage in the cerebellum is not common.

Head injury can be classified into:

1) TRIVIAL INJURY without loss of consciousness and/or posttraumatic amnesia
2) MILD INJURY where the loss of consciousness and/or post traumatic amnesia does not exceed 30 minutes and there is no skull fracture.

3) <u>MODERATE INJURY</u> where loss of consciousness and/or post traumatic amnesia lasts for more than 30 minutes but less than 24 hours and/or a skull fracture is present.

4) <u>SEVERE INJURY</u> where the loss of consciousness and post traumatic amnesia lasts for more than 24 hours and/or cerebral contusion and/or an intracranial haematoma is present.

5) <u>FATAL INJURY,</u> where the patient dies following the head injury.

Categories 3,4,5 are generally accepted as evidence of structural brain damage. Post-traumatic amnesia is the duration for which there is a defect in continuous memory following a head injury. Anterograde amnesia is amnesia for events after the injury. Retrograde amnesia is amnesia for events prior to injury. It is very brief in most cases of head injury and shortens with recovery even in very severe cases.

The Glasgow Coma scale mentioned in chapter 2 could also classify the head injuries. The maximum score in the scale is 15 and minimum is 3. In coma, the scale is around 8 or less. When the scale is around 14-15, the injury is mild, with the scale reading of 9-13 the injury is moderate and the injury is severe, when the coma scale is around 3-8.

Cerebral contusion is a bruise of cerebral tissue following head injury. On CAT scan it appears hypodense with haemorrhagic hyperdense areas. Pathologically there are microhaemorrhages, with loss of neurones and resultant gliosis. Unlike a cerebral infarction the overlying arachnoid membrane undergoes fibrosis as the injury involves the structures from the periphery to the centre. An infarct on the other hand involves areas within a common vascular system, thus sparing the meninges with their external carotid source of blood supply.

The term concussion generally means altered consciousness for a brief period following a mild head injury, but with the amnesia for the event itself. However, it is used rather loosely and has become synonymous with any head injury. It is therefore better not to use the term and classify injury as mentioned above.

Intracranial haematoma includes epidural, subdural and intracerebral haematomas. Where there is collection of CSF instead of blood, the term hygroma is used.

Epidural haemorrhage is an extradural collection of blood generally of arterial origin, usually located in the temporal region due to a tear in the middle meningeal artery. It occurs in about 1 % of an unselected series of head injuries. It is usually biconvex in shape. It is rare under the age of 2 years, as the dura is tightly adherent to the inner table of the skull. A lucid interval after the injury is more often absent than present. A fracture of the temporal bone is invariably present and there may be blood behind the tympanic membrane (Battle's sign). Patient deteriorates rapidly, and constitutes a neurosurgical emergency. Early suspicion offers a better outcome. CAT scan is diagnostic and subtemporal decompression with evacuation of the clot and plugging the middle meningeal leak offers the only chance of saving the patient.

Subdural haematoma is classified as acute, subacute and chronic.

The acute haematoma occurs in the first three days after trauma. They are most common in the first 24-36 hours after the head injury. The acute subdural haematoma occurs in 30 % of severe head injuries. The skull fracture is present in 80 % of cases. The patient shows an increase in focal neurological deficit with deterioration in consciousness. Focal seizures may occur. There is generally underlying brain contusion and even presence of brainstem damage. Intracranial pressure may be raised. The CAT scan gives the diagnosis. The treatment of choice is evacuation by craniotomy. The morbidity and mortality of acute subdural haematoma is very high. The mortality is nearly 70 % for patients over 65 years of age, and few patients are able to lead an independent existence after suffering this severe a head injury.

Subacute subdural haematomas are defined by the existence of a membrane, which is a sprouting of fibroblasts from the inner layer of the dura. It becomes manifest between 4 and 20 days after a head injury. It is otherwise similar to an acute subdural, but has a slightly better outcome.

The chronic subdural haematomas unlike the acute or subacute are found weeks to months after the trauma. The initial injury may be so trivial as to be forgotten. A third of the patients with chronic subdural haematoma do not give any history of trauma. The bleeding is said to be venous in origin, with the formation of crescent shaped clot that compresses the underlying brain. The patient presents with impairment of memory and may even be admitted to a psychiatric unit as a case of organic brain syndrome. The mental status is abnormal with the patient mildly confused and disoriented. There are no focal neurological findings, and the diagnosis may be missed if it is not suspected. Some patients may complain of headache that is worse in the morning and aggravated by coughing and stooping. Seizures are uncommon. A CAT scan makes the diagnosis. The EEG may also be abnormal showing unilateral slowing over the involved area. The haematoma is evacuated by a burr-hole. Multiple tapings may be required. There is good recovery of cognitive functions.

Clinical evaluation of the head injury patient involves ascertaining the occurrence of loss of consciousness and post-traumatic amnesia. Alcohol use in relation to head injury should be noted. Presence of other injuries must be noted and CAT scan done if there is alteration in consciousness after the injury. A neurological surgeon should evaluate patients with rapid deterioration of consciousness and/or focal neurological signs as soon as possible. If on examination patient has unilateral flaccid paralysis, 20 % of these will die. On the other hand if the patient shows decerebration unilaterally or bilaterally then almost 30-60 % will expire. Bilateral flaccid paralysis has the worst prognosis and almost 70 % will die. Any patient with vague history, or with altered mental status, or who complains of sleepiness should be admitted and observed for 24 hours.

The management depends upon the extent of trauma and the presence of fractures and intracranial haematomas. Depressed fractures require surgery and haematomas have to be evacuated. Monitoring the Glasgow Coma scale on an hourly basis or daily and treating increases in intracranial pressure by osmotic agents are important measures in the care of a head injury patient. Severely injured patients need long-term rehabilitation and may be left with substantial cognitive and physical deficit.

INJURIES AT SPECIAL SITES

HYPOTHALAMIC INJURIES produce hyperthermia, with temperature rising above 42 degrees Celsius. Erosion of the gastric mucosa leads to haematemesis. Affection of hypothalamic nuclei produces diabetes insipidus.

BRAINSTEM INJURY is a common secondary feature of severe head injury. Coma, cranial nerve palsies and a poor prognosis are hallmarks of the brainstem involvement

TEMPORAL LOBE is one of the three sites in the brain that have a predilection for developing cerebral contusion. The other two sites are frontal and occipital poles. These are regions where the brain slides and dashes against the uneven bony surface of the anterior and middle cranial fossae. The occipital contusion is usually a contra coupe injury. A temporal lobe contusion can lead to signs of increased intracranial pressure due to oedema of the temporal lobe. Some patients may be dysphasic if the left temporal lobe is involved and others become drowsy and develop unilateral cranial nerve palsy affecting the third and sixth nerves. Carrying out a CAT scan makes the diagnosis of the temporal lobe contusion. The temporal lobe has to be decompressed surgically and contused brain excised.

SPINAL CORD INJURIES

Any injury that is severe enough to cause damage to the spinal cord invariably injures the vertebrae, and the soft tissues such as the ligaments and the muscles. Conversely if the bone and soft tissue are able to withstand the injury, the spinal cord escapes being injured.

Soft tissues such as ligaments and muscles can be injured in hyperextension and hyperflexion that occurs in sudden acceleration or deceleration. Hyperextension is produced by acceleration injuries as when a car is hit from the back by another fast moving vehicle. A head-on collision on the other hand produces sudden deceleration and results in a hyperflexion injury. The symptoms consist of pain at the site of injury and limitation of neck movements. There is usually no associated spinal cord injury. Rarely, hyperextension of the neck leads to a paralysis where the arms are involved to a greater extent then the legs, sensory changes are minimal, and sphincter incontinence may be present.

The treatment of the common whiplash syndrome consists of analgesics and rest with local application of heat and other palliative measures.

Bone injuries leading to dislocation of the vertebrae without fracturing the bone is only possible in the cervical region. The common sites of dislocation are the atlanto-axial joint, and dislocation of C_4 over C_5 or of C_5 over C_6. Atlanto-axial dislocation can cause sudden death due to respiratory paralysis. If the patient survives he may be left with a quadriplegia, with loss of pain and temperature sensation up to the clavicular level, and with marked loss of joint and position sense in the arms. Dislocations at lower levels occur following falls whilst riding or diving into shallow waters. These actions cause excessive flexion of the spine with dislocation at the upper thoracic levels. This results in compression of the spinal cord between the lamina of the upper vertebra and the body of the lower vertebra. Quadriplegia with a sensory loss up to upper thoracic level and with absence of biceps and supinator reflexes may be found. Fracture dislocation is also common at the level of twelfth thoracic and first lumbar vertebrae. Fractures of the spinous and transverse processes and fissures and compression fractures of the lower thoracic vertebral bodies do not lead to neurological complications. Occasionally haematomyelia or extradural haematoma may occur. The extradural haematoma may be evacuated as soon as possible.

In spinal concussion there is a disturbance of the synaptic transmission in the central grey matter, resulting in total paralysis with loss of pain and temperature, both below the level of the lesion, hypotonia, loss of tendon reflexes, and sphincter incontinence. There is preservation of fine touch and proprioceptive sensation, as the posterior columns have no synaptic connections in the spinal cord. There is total recovery of function within 24-48 hours.

Spinal contusion occurs due to nipping of the spinal cord between the lamina of the vertebral body above the lesion and posterior edge of the vertebral body below the lesion. Petechial haemorrhages are widespread in the area. Oedema occurs and haematomyelia may also develop. Clinical features mimic those of a concussion of the cord except that the posterior column is not spared. Sensory level ascends upwards due to increasing oedema. Recovery is poor if not treated early. Spasticity may appear after the recovery of the spinal shock. Haemattomyelia resembles syringomyelia except that the symptomatology is acute in onset.

The aim of therapy is to prevent further injury and one must attempt to realign the vertebral column adequately. Full assessment of the injury by MRI examination is essential. High doses of steroids are used in the form of Methylprednisolone given intravenously. The dose is 30 mg/kg body weight, given in the first 15 minutes. Forty-five minutes later 5.4 mg/kg/hour is given over the next 23 hours. Surgery may be carried out to remove impinged cartilage or bone. Protruded disc tissue should be excised. Nursing care and rehabilitative measures are very important in severely injured cases and play a crucial role in the eventual outcome.

CHAPTER X TUMOURS

Intracranial tumours can be primary, arising from the neuroectodermal tissues or the meninges, or secondary, invading the cranium or intracranial structures due to direct or haematogenous spread. The cause of intracranial tumours is as yet unknown though genetics does play a part and certain viruses such as myxoma virus and chemicals such as tar have been shown to be carcinogenic in animals.

Intracranial tumours can be classified according to their location, cell of origin or growth characteristics. We find the classification used by K.J. Zulch useful and therefore print it in detail below:

Table 10.1

Classification Of Intracranial Tumours

(Modified From The International Histological Classification Of Tumours)

1. **Tumours of Neuroepithelial tissue**
   - A. **Astrocytic tumours:** Astrocytoma, Astroblastoma, Malignant astrocytoma
   - B. **Oligodendroglial tumours:** Oligodendroglioma, Malignant oligodendroglioma
   - C. **Ependymal and choroid plexus tumours:** Ependymoma, Malignant ependymoma, Choroid plexus papiloma, Malignant papiloma.
   - D. **Neuronal tumours:** Gangliocytoma, Ganglioglioma, and Ganglioneuroblastoma, Neuroblastoma.
   - E. **Poorly differentiated and embryonal tumours:** Glioblastoma, Medulloblastoma, Spongioblastoma, Gliomatosis cerebri.
2. **Tumours of Nerve sheath cells**
   - A. Neurilemmoma (Schwanomma, Neurinoma)
   - B. Malignant neurilemmoma

C. Neurofibroma
D. Malignant neurofibroma

3. Tumours of Meningeal and related tissues

A. Meningioma
B. Meningeal sarcoma
C. Xanthomatous tumours (Fibroxanthoma, Xanthosarcoma)
D. Primary Melanotic tumours (Melanoma, Meningeal melanomatosis)

4. Primary Malignant Lymphomas

5. Tumours of blood vessel origin

A. Haemangioblastoma

6. Germ cell tumours

A. Germinoma
B. Embryonal carcinoma
C. Choriocarcinoma
D. Teratoma

7. Other malformative tumours and tumour like lesions

A. Craniopharyngioma
B. Rathke's cleft cyst
C. Epidermoid cyst
D. Dermoid cyst
E. Colloid cyst of the third ventricle
F. Enterogenous cyst
G. Other cysts
H. Lipoma

8. Vascular malformations

A. Capillary telengectasia
B. Cavernous angioma
C. Arterio-venous malformation
D. Venous malformation
E. Sturge-Weber disease (Cerebrotrigeminal angiomatosis)

9. **Tumours of the anterior pituitary**
   A. Pituitary adenoma (Acidophil, Basophil, Mixed and Chromophobe)
   B. Pituitary adenocarcinoma
10. **Local extension from regional tumours**
   A. Glomus jugulare tumour
   B. Chordoma
   C. Chondroma
   D. Chondrosarcoma
   E. Olfactory neuroblastoma
   F. Adenoid cystic carcinoma (Cylindroma)
11. **Metastatic tumours**
12. **Unclassified tumours**

Infective granulomas like tuberculoma, abscesses, and parasitic cysts should not be considered as tumours of the central nervous system, even though they produce signs and symptoms that are akin to tumours. Tumours behave as space occupying lesions, compress important structures, and destroy tissue or destruction and growth occur paripassu as in microgliomas and gliomatosis cerebri.

The clinical features of an intracranial mass depend on its location, its rate of growth and its ability to infiltrate tissue. Cerebral oedema develops with most fast growing tumours and causes further increase in neurological deficit. As the brain is encased in a tight bony compartment of the skull, the tumours do not have much scope for enlargement and before long they cause changes in the sensorium and produce signs of increased intracranial pressure. Some tumours may bleed into its substance causing sudden increase in signs, which mimics a vascular event. Glioblastoma multiforme and oligodendroglioma are the ones, which commonly bleed. The intracranial cavity is further divided into infra and supra tentorial compartments and tumours in either compartment displace structures and lead to signs of herniation. (Figure 10.1)

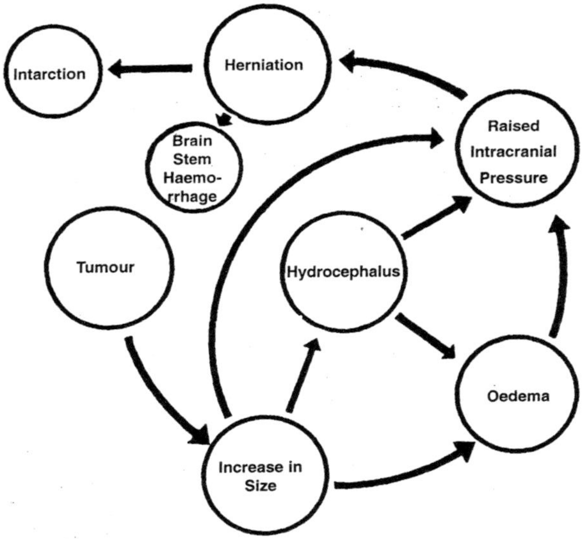

FLOW DIAGRAM SHOWING PROGRESSIVE COMPLICATIONS OF AN INTRACRANIAL TUMOUR

Fig 10.1 Various causes for increased intracranial pressure and herniation

Intracranial pressure is the pressure under which the CSF exists in the cranial cavity. It can be measured by the introduction of a catheter into the lateral ventricle and recording the pressure on an electronic recording apparatus. Modern techniques monitor intracranial pressure continually by the use of transducers that are placed subdurally. Normal intracranial pressure varies between 150-200 mm of CSF. Remember that the brain, the CSF and the blood that flows through this region (normally a fifth of cardiac output), are all contained in a rigid bony cage – the skull – with the foramen magnum providing a small vent for overflow of CSF. Therefore an increase in any three components (Brain, CSF, blood) must result in displacement of the other two. Small and gradual rises in intracranial pressure can be accommodated without any significant effects, but sudden and large increases in pressure are dangerous and can prove fatal if remedial measures are not taken on an emergency basis. These effects are due to the result of brainstem dysfunction that occurs due to the rostro-caudal displacement of the contents of the supratentorial compartment. Depending on the site of the lesion responsible for these events, first the cingulate gyrus herniates under the falx, then the uncus of the temporal lobe herniates under the tentorium and finally the medulla herniates through the foramen magnum.(Fig 10.2) Increase in CSF pressure alone does not lead to herniation, as in pseudo tumour cerebri, but any event that causes obstruction to the flow of arterial blood or spinal fluid begins the process. Arterial blood continues to be pumped in, accelerating the herniation, till intracranial pressure rises above that of arterial pressure. When this occurs there is no intracranial blood flow, a sign that can be demonstrated on angiography and constitutes one of the tests for documenting brain death.

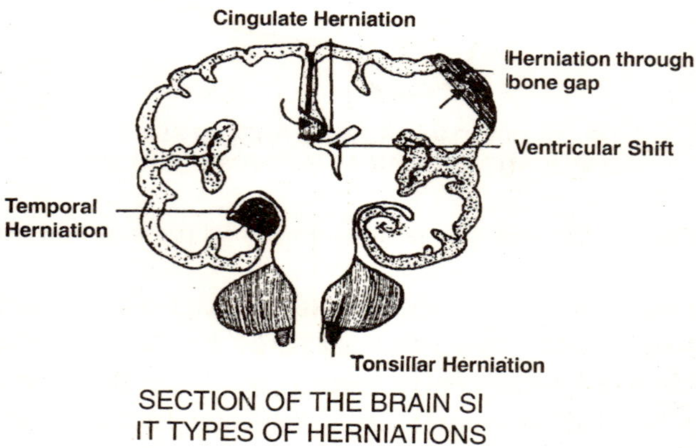

Fig 10.2 Coronal section of the brain showing different types of herniation

Causes of intracranial pressure are legion. Besides tumours they include a) haematoma: extradural, subdural and intracerebral, b) acqueductal stenosis, c) intracranial abscess and granulomas d) obstructive hydrocephalus.

The symptoms of increased intracranial pressure include headache, drowsiness and blurring of vision. The headache is of moderate severity and can be associated with projectile vomiting. Since this vomiting is central in origin, there is no preceding nausea. Further increase in pressure causes changes in the level of consciousness with the patient becoming drowsy. The brainstem is compressed and pathologically shows small haemorrhages known as "duret" haemorrhages. Pupillary changes have been described previously and will not be repeated here but one must bear in mind that an ipsilateral large pupil that does not react to light may be found.

Some intracranial tumours are associated with change in personality. The patient becomes placid and withdrawn or hyperexcitable. The ability to concentrate suffers ands there is loss of recent memory. Seizures may occur due to focal brain involvement. Partial seizures are common in gliomas and granulomas. Focal seizures that begin after the age of twenty are more likely due to tumours. In fact in some series the incidence is reported to be as high as 10 %.

TUMOURS OF THE FRONTAL LOBE

Loss of initiative, placidity and apathy may be the presenting features of a frontal lobe tumour. Sometimes the patient may demonstrate a silly sense of humour, with a tendency to use puns, the so-called "witzelsucht" that is due to loss of frontal inhibition. The patient may loose his job, because of lack of interest and concentration; he may become unconcerned about his dress and personal appearance and may even be euphoric. Seizures are common with frontal lobe tumours and may be focal motor or adversive in type. An adversive seizure consists of head and eyes turning opposite to the side of discharge and on some occasions progressing to a generalised seizure.

Except for dementia and an abnormal affect, there may be few physical signs to demonstrate. A grasp reflex may be present. The examiner clasps the patient's hand and then lets it go suddenly. If the grasp reflex is present the patient involuntarily grasps the examiner's fingers. A bilateral grasp reflex has no localising value, but a unilateral grasp reflex points to contralateral frontal lobe pathology. Tumours that infiltrate the motor strip lead to contralateral motor signs that vary from a mild weakness of the lower limb to a hemiparesis. A lesion that affects the speech area causes disturbance in speech. A parasagittal tumour causes bilateral weakness and sphincter symptoms due to involvement of the paracentral lobule.

There may be mild facial weakness with some frontal tumours as the face area is more anterior than the arm and leg. False localising signs occur when a cerebellar tumour causes hydrocephalus and the frontal lobe is subject to increased pressure. Signs of frontal lobe involvement may then lead to faulty localisation. Tumours of the orbital surface of the frontal lobe may grow to a considerable size before causing symptoms.

TUMOURS OF THE PARIETAL LOBE

The parietal lobe contains the sensory cortex; hence tumours in this region cause sensory seizures that consist of paraesthesias in the opposite half of the body. Lesions of the dominant parietal lobe cause the "Gerstmann syndrome" with agraphia, finger agnosia, acalculia, astereognosis and loss of two-point discrimination. Non-dominant parietal lobe tumours lead to dressing apraxia, loss of body image and loss of topographical memory.

Sensory inattention is the inability to recognise stimuli on one half of the body. When both sides of the body are touched simultaneously, the patient cannot recognise stimuli on the affected side. Involvement of the visual association areas lead to visual inattention, with the patient tending to bump into objects in the affected visual field and inability to perform motor action in the presence of normal muscle strength. Apraxia is also a feature of parietal lobe lesion.

TUMOURS OF THE OCCIPITAL LOBE

Tumours can destroy the visual cortex or affect the visual association areas. Seizures presenting as simple visual hallucinations, are seen in posteriorly located tumours. Flashes of light, coloured lights and circles of light may be reported in the involved visual field. A hemianopia is a common defect in occipital lobe lesions, though altitudinal defects have also been observed. When the occipital pole is spared, hemianopia with spared macular vision is noted.

TUMOURS OF THE TEMPORAL LOBE

The temporal lobe is the most complex lobe of the brain. Rolled up in a manner of a scroll, encased in the narrow confines of the middle cranial fossa, it is difficult for the student to visualise, as compared to the other lobes, which are relatively simple. Not only does a region of the temporal lobe such as hippocampus have different blood supply, but also within the same area there is different vulnerability to lack of oxygen. The temporal lobe is also diverse in its function; it plays a role in emotional, motor and autonomic activity. Therefore it is not surprising that tumours of the temporal lobe may present in many different ways. Lesions that involve the anterior temporal lobe result in 'psychomotor' seizures. Other temporal lobe lesions may cause disturbances in cognition, or dysamnestic symptoms like 'jamais vu or déjà vu'. Déjà vu is a feeling of familiarity with an unfamiliar situation, whilst jamais vu is the sensation of feeling strange in a familiar surrounding. Hallucination of taste, smell, and vision may occur depending on the site of the tumour. Disturbances in affect such as spells of intense fear or depression have been reported. Seizures that consist of automatism are common with the automatism involving the face and specially the lips or tongue. If the Meyer's loop is involved a superior quadrantic defect may be demonstrated. Problems with memory may be a prominent feature in lesions that involve the hippocampal region. Rarely sexual disturbances may occur.

TUMOURS OF THE BRAIN STEM

The brain stem consists of three parts: the midbrain, the pons and the medulla. The corticospinal fibres descend via the cerebral peduncles and then through the basis pontis before decussating in the medulla. Fibres are so arranged in the midbrain that fibres meant for the leg lie most laterally, while fibres for the arm are located more medially. Fibres supplying the motor nuclei of various cranial nerves are most medial in location. The sensory tracts unite in the midbrain and lie anterior to the nucleus of the third nerve. In the pons the medial lemniscus is located somewhat laterally in the corpus trapezoidum. The spino-thalamic tract lies postero-laterally in relation to the medial lemniscus. In the medulla, gracile nucleus is medial and the cuneate nucleus lies just lateral to it. Nuclei of the cranial nerves are generally located dorsal to the ascending and descending pathways.

The commonest tumour of the brainstem is a glioma that occurs more frequently in children and is very slow growing. In India a tuberculoma is equally likely, causing some neurosurgeons to treat a 'brainstem tumour' with antituberculous therapy before considering a neoplastic lesion.

A brainstem glioma causes sixth and seventh nerve weakness, with the child showing signs of diplopia and facial weakness. Signs of pyramidal tract involvement such as spasticity and hyperreflexia are present though frank paralysis occurs late in the course of the disease. As the tumour grows ataxia may appear. Sensory signs are however rare and occur only in about a fifth of patients. Though vomiting may result from medullary involvement, headaches are uncommon, as hydrocephalus does not occur till very late in the course of illness.

TUMOURS OF THE PITUITARY GLAND

These tumours lie in the close proximity of the optic chiasm and cause bitemporal or binasal hemianopia. Optic atrophy occurs frequently and papilloedema has also been reported. Disturbances of endocrine function like gigantism, acromegaly or Cushing's disease may occur. The most common pituitary tumour of childhood is the craniopharyngioma whilst the chromophobe adenoma occurs in older individuals. Rise of prolactin levels and disturbances of fertility can occur due to microadenoma of the pituitary gland.

TUMOURS OF THE PINEAL BODY

"Parinaud's syndrome", a paralysis of the upward gaze is common with the tumours of the pineal body. A mild bilateral ptosis, dilated pupils and sluggish or even absent pupillary light reflex may be observed. Tumours in this region lead to rapid development of hydrocephalus and changes in the level of consciousness. Precocious puberty has been reported in pineal tumours.

TUMOURS OF THE THALAMUS AND BASAL GANGLIA

These tumours produce personality changes, and signs of extrapyramidal involvement such as parkinsonism, choreoathetosis and dystonia. Hemiparesis is seen due to involvement of the adjacent internal capsule.

TUMOURS OF THE EIGHTH NERVE

These tumours have already been described under the discussion of the eighth cranial nerve. A few additional features are mentioned here. The acoustic neurinoma comprises about 8 % of all intracranial tumours and 80 % of all tumours in the cerebellopontine angle. There is 2:1 preponderance in females as compared to males. Symptoms of cranial nerve involvement occur early where as symptoms of increased intracranial pressure occur very late in the disease.

TUMOURS OF THE CEREBELLUM

These tumours can occur at any age, but the medulloblastoma – a malignant tumour in the region of vermis, and astrocytoma of the cerebellar hemisphere are more common in the childhood. Haemangioma may form a part of the Phakomatosis (von Hippel Landau" disease). Cerebellar tumours cause ataxia and in the case of medulloblastoma, vomiting with rapid signs of increased intracranial pressure with papilloedema and hydrocephalus are noted. On examination, signs of cerebellar disease such as titubation, hypotonia, dysmetria and nystagmus are seen.

COLLOID CYST OF THE THIRD VENTRICLE

These cysts are mobile and can occlude the foramen of Monro and the aqueduct of Sylvius suddenly leading to signs and symptoms of hydrocephalus. Intermittent obstruction of the foramina of Monro results in severe paroxysmal headache, which is relieved by a change in position of the head. These tumours can also cause sudden death. Other signs of third ventricular involvement like somnolence, polyuria, obesity, loss of libido are rare with colloid cyst but occur with third ventricular glioma.

DIFFERENTIAL DIAGNOSIS OF AN INTRACRANIAL MASS:

An intracranial abscess or a granuloma is the most important differential diagnosis that should be considered. Abscesses tend to be located in the temporal lobe or cerebellum when they occur due to direct spread of the infection from the inner ear. Abscesses that are secondary to haematogenous spread are usually located in the parietal lobes. Frontal lobe abscesses are likely to be the result of an extension of infection in the frontal or ethmoidal sinuses. The presentation of an abscess can be either acute or chronic. Acute lesions cause mild fever with leucocytosis. Signs of cerebritis and meningeal irritation may be present. There may be a history of ear discharge, or sinus infection. Chronic abscesses may sometimes only be diagnosed at surgery. Papilloedema occurs late with abscesses but there may be widespread cerebral oedema.

Tuberculomas are a common cause of space occupying lesions in our country and also in patients with AIDS. In children they tend to be located in the posterior fossa. After the age of twenty they are usually supratentorial in location. Presence of tuberculosis elsewhere in the body, a positive Mantoux test and an elevated ESR should raise the suspicion of tuberculoma. Presence of HIV infection should also raise the suspicion of either tuberculoma or granuloma due to toxoplasma or fungal granuloma. If the patient's visual deficit or clinical status is not grave enough to warrant immediate surgery, it is preferable to try antituberculous therapy or medical management of the granuloma with antibiotics prior to surgery. Sometimes a biopsy under stereotaxic control should be carried out to ascertain the nature of the granuloma.

Congenital lesion such as aqueductal stenosis, the Chiari malformation and the Dandy-Walker syndrome may be mistaken for a tumour if the course is atypical. Hypertensive encephalopathy leads to sudden change in sensorium, focal neurological deficit and seizures. The symptoms subside when the blood pressure is brought under control. Chronic subdural haematoma is another possibility, especially in the elderly. They present with history of gradual mental deterioration, diminished alertness and lucidity.

Psuedotumour cerebri is a diagnosis of exclusion and is found to occur in young obese females. There is history of headaches and blurring of vision. The blind spot is enlarged; there is bilateral papilloedema but no focal neurological deficit. Sometimes there is history of menstrual disorder or of use of oral contraceptives. This condition is also known as benign intracranial hypertension. Also, cerebral venous sinus obstruction should be ruled out if there is a history of ear discharge or use of oral contraceptive. Cerebral vein thrombosis usually presents with seizures, focal or generalised and focal signs with signs of increased intracranial pressure.

In India, psuedotumour cerebri like presentation can be secondary to cysticercosis. Cysticercosis can also present with seizures, focal or generalised. Vitamin A intoxication and polycythemia are rare causes of pseudotumour cerebri. All laboratory tests including EEG and CAT scan are normal. Very small slit like ventricles have been described with pseudotumour, but they can be seen in normal young people. Efacement of gyri and sulci may be seen in pseudotumour.

The presence of an intracranial neoplasm or mass should be suspected in any patient who gives a history of progressive increase in focal neurological symptoms such as weakness of a limb, a history of partial seizures occurring mainly in sleep. The course is very short with a malignant lesion, but can be very gradual with acoustic neurinoma and brainstem glioma.

EEG may be helpful at times in suspecting an intracranial mass. It is abnormal in 70 % of cases with hemispheric tumours and tends to be normal or shows mild generalised abnormality in cases of posterior fossa lesions. It is usually normal in deep-seated hemispheric tumours.

CAT scan with contrast enhancement and plain MRI and at times with gadolinium enhancement will help in arriving at a conclusive diagnosis. Rarely cerebral angiography is indicated.

MANAGEMENT OF AN INTRACRANIAL MASS

It consists of two parts, one, treating the intracranial pressure and second, treating the causative lesion.

MANAGEMENT OF INCREASED INTRACRANIAL PRESSURE

Cerebral oedema is best defined as an increase in brain volume that is due to an increase in its water content. Brain oedema is of three types: Vasogenic, Cytotoxic and Interstitial. Intracranial tumours are associated with vasogenic oedema. Vasogenic oedema is caused by an increase in capillary permeability and is chiefly localised in the white matter. The oedema fluid consists of plasma filtrate including plasma proteins. This type of oedema responds to therapy with steroids and responds to osmotic agents. Acetazolamide and Frusemide are of questionable value. Dexamethasone is given daily in divided doses of 12-16 mg intravenously. Mannitol is very useful osmotic agent. Twenty per cent of mannitol in a 300 ml solution is administered over 3-4 hours intravenously, which reduces the intracranial pressure acutely. The longer duration of administration is preferable to avoid a rebound rise in pressure, compared to rapid administration. Subtemporal decompression of ventriculo-atrial or peritoneal shunt procedures are necessary in life threatening situations and in cases where cerebral oedema is refractory to medical management.

Management of tumour mass depends on the nature and location of the tumour. Ideally the tumour should be resected in toto. Some tumours are radiosensitive and respond well to radiation. If malignant, the resection is followed by radiation and chemotherapy.

INDEX

B

N